COMPREHENSIVE BIOCHEMISTRY

ELSEVIER PUBLISHING COMPANY
335 Jan van Galenstraat, P.O. Box 211, Amsterdam, The Netherlands

ELSEVIER PUBLISHING COMPANY LIMITED
Barking, Essex, England

AMERICAN ELSEVIER PUBLISHING COMPANY, INC.
52 Vanderbilt Avenue, New York, N.Y. 10017

Library of Congress Card Number 62–10359
ISBN 0-444-40950-5

With 20 illustrations and 11 tables

COMPREHENSIVE BIOCHEMISTRY

COMPREHENSIVE BIOCHEMISTRY

SECTION I (VOLUMES 1–4)
PHYSICO-CHEMICAL AND ORGANIC ASPECTS
OF BIOCHEMISTRY

SECTION II (VOLUMES 5–11)
CHEMISTRY OF BIOLOGICAL COMPOUNDS

SECTION III (VOLUMES 12–16)
BIOCHEMICAL REACTION MECHANISMS

SECTION IV (VOLUMES 17–21)
METABOLISM

SECTION V (VOLUMES 22–29)
CHEMICAL BIOLOGY

HISTORY OF BIOCHEMISTRY (VOLUME 30)

GENERAL INDEX (VOLUME 31)

COMPREHENSIVE
BIOCHEMISTRY

EDITED BY

MARCEL FLORKIN

Professor of Biochemistry, University of Liège (Belgium)

AND

ELMER H. STOTZ

Professor of Biochemistry, University of Rochester, School of Medicine and Dentistry, Rochester, N.Y. (U.S.A.)

VOLUME 18S

PYRUVATE AND FATTY ACID METABOLISM

ELSEVIER PUBLISHING COMPANY

AMSTERDAM · LONDON · NEW YORK

1971

CONTRIBUTORS TO THIS VOLUME

EUGENE M. BARNES JR., PH.D.
Research Associate, Department of Biochemistry, Duke University Medical Center,
Durham, N.C. 27706 (U.S.A.)

JOHN M. LOWENSTEIN, B.SC., PH.D.
Professor of Biochemistry, Graduate Department of Biochemistry, Brandeis
University, Waltham, Mass. 02154 (U.S.A.)

SALIH J. WAKIL
Professor of Biochemistry, Department of Biochemistry, Duke University Medical
Center, Durham, N.C. 27706 (U.S.A.)

GENERAL PREFACE

The Editors are keenly aware that the literature of Biochemistry is already very large, in fact so widespread that it is increasingly difficult to assemble the most pertinent material in a given area. Beyond the ordinary textbook the subject matter of the rapidly expanding knowledge of biochemistry is spread among innumerable journals, monographs, and series of reviews. The Editors believe that there is a real place for an advanced treatise in biochemistry which assembles the principal areas of the subject in a single set of books.

It would be ideal if an individual or small group of biochemists could produce such an advanced treatise, and within the time to keep reasonably abreast of rapid advances, but this is at least difficult if not impossible. Instead, the Editors with the advice of the Advisory Board, have assembled what they consider the best possible sequence of chapters written by competent authors; they must take the responsibility for inevitable gaps of subject matter and duplication which may result from this procedure.

Most evident to the modern biochemists, apart from the body of knowledge of the chemistry and metabolism of biological substances, is the extent to which he must draw from recent concepts of physical and organic chemistry, and in turn project into the vast field of biology. Thus in the organization of Comprehensive Biochemistry, the middle three sections, Chemistry of Biological Compounds, Biochemical Reaction Mechanisms, and Metabolism may be considered classical biochemistry, while the first and last sections provide selected material on the origins and projections of the subject.

It is hoped that sub-division of the sections into bound volumes will not only be convenient, but will find favour among students concerned with specialized areas, and will permit easier future revisions of the individual volumes. Toward the latter end particularly, the Editors will welcome all comments in their effort to produce a useful and efficient source of biochemical knowledge.

M. FLORKIN
E. H. STOTZ

Liège/Rochester

PREFACE TO SECTION IV

(VOLUMES 17–21)

Metabolism in its broadest context may be regarded as the most dynamic aspect of biochemistry, yet depends entirely for its advances on progress in the knowledge of the structure of natural compounds, structure–function relationships in enzymes, bioenergetics, and cytochemistry. Approaches to the study of metabolism range from whole organism studies, with limited possibility to reveal mechanisms, to cytochemical or even purified enzyme systems, sometimes with little attention to physiological conditions. Yet all approaches broaden our understanding of metabolism, and all of them may be recognized in the volumes assembled in Section IV on *Metabolism*. It is not unexpected then that previous sections of *Comprehensive Biochemistry* actually deal with some aspects under the broad heading of *Metabolism*, and certainly that the succeeding Section V on *Chemical Biology* should draw heavily on basic understanding of metabolism. Nevertheless Section IV attempts to bring together the broad outlines of the metabolism of amino acids, proteins, carbohydrates, lipids, and their derived products. The currently rapid advances in feed-back, hormonal, and genetic control of metabolism make it particularly difficult that these volumes be current, but the authors, editors, and publishers have made all possible efforts to include the most recent advances.

This supplementary volume to Section IV on *Metabolism* contains two essential chapters which were not available to the Editors earlier. The first, entitled "The Pyruvate Dehydrogenase Complex and the Citric Acid Cycle" by J. M. Lowenstein was originally planned for Volume 17 on *Carbohydrate Metabolism*, and the second, entitled "Fatty Acid Metabolism" by Salih J. Wakil and E. M. Barnes Jr., was planned for Volume 18 on *Lipid Metabolism*.

Liège/Rochester

M. FLORKIN
E. H. STOTZ

CONTENTS

VOLUME 18S

PYRUVATE AND FATTY ACID METABOLISM

Chapter I. The Pyruvate Dehydrogenase Complex and the Citric Acid Cycle

by J. M. LOWENSTEIN

Chapter II. Fatty Acid Metabolism

by SALIH J. WAKIL AND EUGENE M. BARNES JR.

Chapter I

The Pyruvate Dehydrogenase Complex and the Citric Acid Cycle

J. M. LOWENSTEIN

Graduate Department of Biochemistry, Brandeis University, Waltham, Mass. (U.S.A.)

1. Pyruvate dehydrogenase

(a) Mechanism

The oxidative decarboxylation of pyruvate to acetyl-coenzyme A occurs according to the following reaction sequence (where TPP is thiamine pyrophosphate):

$$\text{Pyruvate} + \text{TPP} \rightarrow \text{1-hydroxyethyl-TPP} + CO_2 \tag{1}$$
$$\text{1-Hydroxyethyl-TPP} + \text{lipoic acid}_{oxid.} \rightarrow \text{acetyllipoic acid}_{red.} + \text{TPP} \tag{2}$$
$$\text{Acetyllipoic acid}_{red.} + HS \cdot CoA \rightarrow \text{acetyl} \cdot S \cdot CoA + \text{lipoic acid}_{red.} \tag{3}$$
$$\text{Lipoic acid}_{red.} + NAD^+ \rightarrow \text{lipoic acid}_{oxid.} + NADH + H^+ \tag{4}$$

Sum:
$$\text{Pyruvate} + HS \cdot CoA + NAD^+ \rightarrow \text{acetyl} \cdot S \cdot CoA + CO_2 + NADH + H^+ \tag{5}$$

These reactions represent the mechanism of pyruvate oxidation in animal tissues and in many microorganisms. The sequence, which was discovered during the early nineteen fifties[1-8], consists of at least four steps and involves five different cofactors, namely thiamine pyrophosphate (TPP), lipoid acid, coenzyme A, FAD, and NAD. The four steps are catalyzed by an enzyme complex which has been highly purified from a variety of sources.

(i) Pyruvate decarboxylase

This member of the pyruvate dehydrogenase complex catalyzes the reaction

[1]

between pyruvate and TPP, which results in the decarboxylation of pyruvate and the formation of the intermediate 1-hydroxyethyl-TPP (reaction 6).

$$
\begin{array}{c}
\text{COOH} \\
| \\
\text{CO} \\
| \\
\text{CH}_3
\end{array}
+ \text{TPP} \leftrightarrow
\begin{array}{c}
\text{CHO[TPP]} \\
| \\
\text{CH}_3
\end{array}
+ \text{CO}_2
\qquad (6)
$$

Evidence in support of this formulation includes the observation that TPP is required for the exchange of $^{14}CO_2$ into pyruvate which is catalyzed by preparations of pyruvate dehydrogenase from pig heart. The exchange reaction does not require coenzyme A and NAD[9-11]. It is not inhibited by arsenite, which indicates that dihydrolipoic acid is not involved[12]. Moreover, pyruvate decarboxylase obtained by resolution of the pyruvate dehydrogenase complex from *Escherichia coli*, which catalyzes reaction 2, does not contain lipoic acid[13]. The mammalian and the bacterial pyruvate dehydrogenase complexes, as well as pyruvate decarboxylase derived from the complex, catalyze pyruvate oxidation in the presence of ferricyanide as electron acceptor. This reaction requires TPP but occurs in the absence of CoA and NAD[2,4,14,15]. The acyl acceptor is water, and the product is acetate. Similar results have been obtained in studies of α-ketoglutarate oxidation linked to ferricyanide reduction[3,15].

The initial step of reaction 1 involves the addition of pyruvate to the

(7)

2'-position of TPP. This is followed by the decarboxylation reaction, the product being 2'-(1-hydroxyethyl)-TPP[17-20]. Both the pyruvate adduct of

$$+ CO_2 \qquad\qquad (8)$$

TPP and hydroxyethyl-TPP have been isolated from incubation mixtures containing pyruvate and pyruvate dehydrogenase[21,22]. Synthetic hydroxyethyl-TPP gives rise to acetyl-coenzyme A when it is incubated with pyruvate dehydrogenase, NAD and coenzyme A[23]. This reaction is much slower than the overall reaction with pyruvate[24], but this does not necessarily argue against the participation of hydroxyethyl-TPP. The hydrogen atom on the 2'-carbon of TPP is particularly labile, and exchanges non-enzymatically with labeled hydrogen from water[17,25]. The rate of non-enzymatic hydrogen exchange at the 2'-position is increased by magnesium ions[26], which are also required for the enzymatic reaction.

(ii) Lipoyl reductase

This enzyme catalyzes the transfer of the hydroxyethyl group from hydroxyethyl-TPP to lipoic acid. In the course of the transfer reaction the hydroxyethyl group is oxidized to an acetyl group with the concomitant reduction of the lipoate to dihydrolipoate. The products are enzyme-bound 6-*S*-acetyldihydrolipoate and TPP. The process can be imagined to be initiated by the removal of a proton from hydroxyethyl-TPP, which then reacts with lipoate as follows:

$$(9)$$

To complete the reaction the TPP–carbanion is protonated to yield TPP.

This stage does not involve coenzyme A, since it has been found that the analogous reaction with α-ketoglutarate yields a succinyl derivative which readily forms succinomonohydroxamate in the presence of hydroxylamine and in the complete absence of coenzyme A[27]. The inhibition of pyruvate and α-ketoglutarate oxidation by arsenite is additional evidence for the involvement of acyl dihydrolipoate in this process[8,27]. The arsenite inhibition requires α-ketoacid to generate acyl dihydrolipoate, and coenzyme A to convert the acyl-dihydrolipoate to dihydrolipoate. The latter is then rendered inactive by reaction with arsenite to form a stable cyclic thioarsenite[28].

The lipoic acid is covalently bound to the enzyme[5,8,14,29-32]. In the case of the bacterial enzyme, the carboxyl group of lipoic acid is in an amide linkage with an ε-amino group of a lysine residue[32]. Work with the pyruvate dehydrogenase complex has failed to demonstrate the occurrence of free acetyl-dihydrolipoate. No exchange between added lipoate and enzyme-bound lipoate could be observed[31,32]. For further details on the chemistry and function of lipoic acid the reader is referred to the special chapter on this topic[8].

(iii) Acetyl transferase

The enzyme catalyzes the transfer of the acetyl group from the thiol group of dihydrolipoate to the thiol group of coenzyme A. The products are dihydrolipoate and acetyl-coenzyme A[33]:

(10)

Reversibility of the reaction can be demonstrated with added dihydrolipoic acid using an acetyl-coenzyme A generating system consisting of acetyl phosphate and coenzyme A[4]. The natural isomer, (−)-lipoate, is acetylated much faster than (+)-lipoate[8]. The product of the reverse reaction is 6-S-acetyllipoate[33].

(iv) Dihydrolipoate dehydrogenase[8]

The enzyme has been highly purified[13,34] and separated from other members of α-ketoacid dehydrogenase complexes. It contains FAD, and catalyzes the reversible oxidation of dihydrolipoate to lipoate using NAD as hydrogen acceptor (reaction 4). Free dihydrolipoate and lipoate serve as substrates for the pig-heart enzyme[35]. However, as has already been stated, in the pyruvate dehydrogenase complex the carboxyl group of lipoate exists as an amide with ε-amino groups of lysine residues of lipoyl reductase.

Dihydrolipoate dehydrogenase possesses a reactive disulfide which participates in the oxidation reaction. The overall dehydrogenase reaction (4) involves a transfer of two electrons from dihydrolipoate to NAD. Spectral evidence indicates that a biradical, comprising a flavin semiquinone and possibly a sulfide radical (R–S ·) are involved in the electron-transfer reaction[36,37]. The enzyme is inhibited by arsenite and by cadmium ions provided NADH is present. The inhibition is reversed readily by BAL (British Antilewisite) and also by monothiols[14,27,38,39]. Addition to the enzyme of NADH results in the appearance of two additional sulfhydryl groups per mole of flavin, suggesting that a disulfide is reduced by this treatment which is then susceptible to arsenite inhibition[39,40].

Straub's diaphorase[41], an enzyme preparation capable of oxidizing NADH in the presence of certain artificial electron acceptors, and dihydrolipoate dehydrogenase have been demonstrated to be the same enzyme[16,42,43]. For further details the reader is referred to the special article by Reed[8] elsewhere in this series, and to the review by Massey[7].

(v) Molecular architecture[44,45]

The pyruvate dehydrogenase complex from E. coli has been isolated in pure form and possesses a molecular weight of about 4.8 million (refs. 44,46). It has been resolved into three separate enzymes, namely pyruvate decarboxylase, lipoyl reductase–acetyl transferase, and dihydrolipoate dehydrogenase. The complex can be reconstituted by combining the separate enzymes[13]. Lipoyl reductase–acetyl transferase can be separated further into two enzymes by calcium phosphate gel chromatography at pH 9.5.

The component enzymes occur in the complex in the following proportions: pyruvate decarboxylase, 12 molecules of molecular weight 183 000; lipoyl reductase–acetyl transferase, 24 subunits of molecular weight 70 000; and dihydrolipoate dehydrogenase, 6 molecules of molecular weight 112 000 (ref. 44). The total molecular weight calculated from these figures is 4.6 million. Dihydrolipoate dehydrogenase contains two moles of FAD per mole of enzyme[13], or twelve moles of FAD per mole of native dehydrogenase complex. Lipoyl reductase–acetyl transferase contains approximately one lipoic acid residue per 35 000 g of protein, or 48 residues per mole of the enzyme or of the native dehydrogenase complex. Treatment with acetic acid at pH 2.6 dissociates lipoyl reductase–acetyl transferase into inactive subunits possessing a molecular weight of 70 000. Rapid dilution of these subunits into buffer at pH 7.0 leads to restoration of enzymatic activity[44,47]. Attempts at partial reconstitution show that pyruvate decarboxylase and dihydrolipoate dehydrogenase do not combine with each other. However, either of these enzymes combines with lipoyl reductase–acetyl transferase[13,44]. When all three are mixed together, a pyruvate dehydrogenase complex is produced which is similar to the native complex.

Electron micrographs of the pyruvate dehydrogenase complex, of lipoyl reductase–acetyl transferase, of the pyruvate dehydrogenase component, and of dihydrolipoate dehydrogenase, prepared from *E. coli*, show that the enzymes of the complex are assembled in an orderly array with a diameter of 300–350 Å (Fig. 1). Phosphotungstate-stained preparations of the whole complex show a polyhedral structure in the center of which can be seen a tetrameric arrangement of subunits. The latter appears to be square when viewed end-on. The tetrameric center is symmetrically surrounded by twelve further subunits which are 60–90 Å in diameter. The outer subunits appear to be organized in the form of staggered rings, although other, more complex, arrangements cannot be ruled out at present.

Preparations of lipoyl reductase–acetyl transferase negatively stained with phosphotungstate reveal tetramers which closely resemble those seen in the center of the pyruvate dehydrogenase complex (Fig. 2). The sides of the tetramers measure 120–140 Å approximately. In addition to the square tetramers, some molecules appear as two parallel strands which are more than two subunits in length. A few appear more complex, possibly in the shape of hexagons. Reed and co-workers[44,45,47] interpret these pictures as indicating that the subunits are arranged into cubes consisting of two tetramers which appear as squares when viewed end-on, as parallel strands when viewed with one edge towards the viewer, and as hexagons when viewed with one corner towards the viewer.

Preparations of the pyruvate dehydrogenase component of the complex show a variety of images under the electron microscope which suggest this component consists of a tetrahedral arrangement of four subunits. Recent studies indicate that these subunits are composed of two pairs of different polypeptide chains, each with a molecular weight of about 45 000 (ref. 45).

A tentative model of the whole complex which is based on the electron micrographs just discussed is shown in Fig. 3. The complex has a relatively "open" structure, in agreement with electron micrographs and with its hydrodynamic characteristics which show a high ratio of frictional coefficients (f/f_o about 1.6) and a low axial ratio (less than 2 to 1).

The highly purified pyruvate dehydrogenase complex from pigeon breast muscle possesses a molecular weight of about $4 \cdot 10^6$ (refs. 48, 49). No further work appears to have been carried out with this preparation since the early nineteen fifties. Most subsequent work has been concerned with the

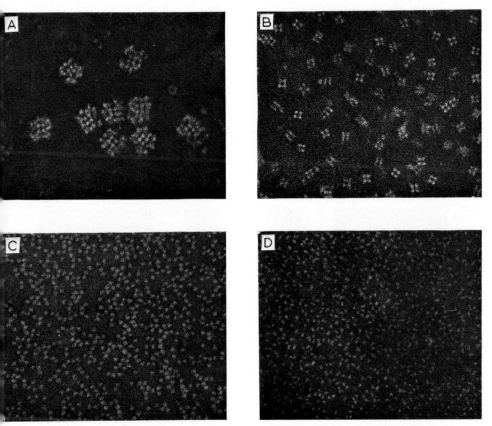

Fig. 1. Pyruvate dehydrogenase complex from *E. coli*, and its components. Electron micrographs ($\times$ 200000) were taken of preparations which had been stained negatively with phosphotungstate. *A*, Pyruvate dehydrogenase complex; *B*, lipoyl reductase–acetyl transferase; *C*, pyruvate dehydrogenase; and *D*, dihydrolipoate dehydrogenase. Reproduced by permission of Reed and Oliver[45] and Brookhaven Laboratories.

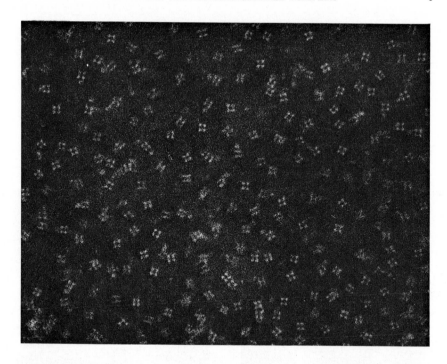

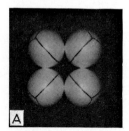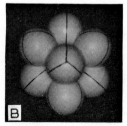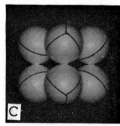

Fig. 2. Lipoyl reductase–transacetylase from *E. coli* ($\times$ 200 000). Also shown are models of the enzyme consisting of eight spheres arranged as a cube, viewed: *A*, side-on; *B*, corner-on; and *C*, edge-on. The black lines are intended to represent the division of each sphere into the three identical chains comprising the subunits of the enzyme. Reproduced by permission of Reed and Oliver[45] and Brookhaven Laboratories.

pyruvate dehydrogenase complex isolated from pig heart and beef kidney. The pig-heart complex possesses a molecular weight of about $9 \cdot 10^6$ (ref. 50).

The complexes from beef kidney[51] and pig heart[50,52] have been resolved into 3 components consisting of pyruvate decarboxylase, lipoyl reductase–

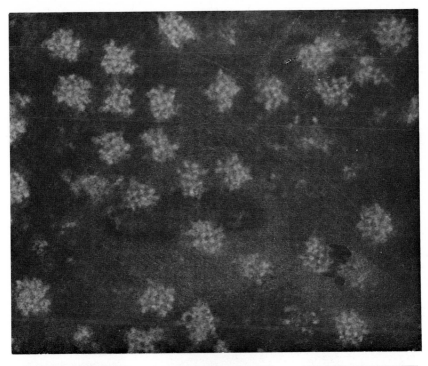

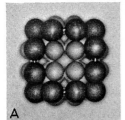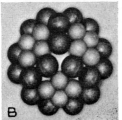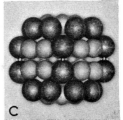

Fig. 3. Electron micrograph of pyruvate dehydrogenase complex ($\times$ 300000), and various interpretative models of the complex viewed down: *A*, a 4-fold axis; *B*, a 3-fold axis; and *C*, a 2-fold axis of symmetry. 24 pyruvate dehydrogenase units (black) and 24 dihydroli-poate dehydrogenase units (white) are placed in a symmetrical manner around a lipoyl reductase–acetyl transferase cube. Reproduced by permission of Reed and Oliver[45] and Brookhaven Laboratories.

acetyl transferase, and dihydrolipoate dehydrogenase[51,53]. Each mole of the enzyme complex isolated from pig heart contains approximately 30 moles of protein-bound lipoic acid and 14 moles of bound FAD, but it is free of TPP[53].

Electron micrographs of lipoyl reductase–transacetylase from beef kidney show an arrangement of subunits quite different from that seen with the same enzyme from *E. coli* (Fig. 4 A)[44,45]. The kidney enzyme appears as a polyhedron with a diameter of about 210 Å. A model which fits the various profiles discernible in the electron micrographs is shown in Fig. 4 A, B and C. Reed and Cox[44] speculate that pyruvate decarboxylase and lipoyl dehydrogenase must be grouped around this polyhedron in the intact pyruvate dehydrogenase complex.

The molecular architecture of the pyruvate dehydrogenase complex was elucidated by combining the techniques of enzymology and molecular electron microscopy. Although many details of structure and mechanism remain to be worked out, this work constitutes one of the landmarks of modern biochemistry.

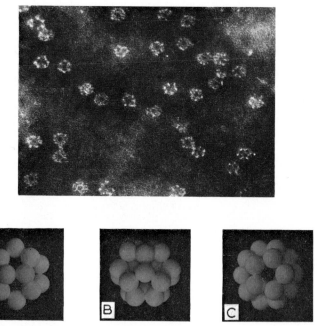

Fig. 4. Lipoyl reductase–acetyl transferase prepared from the mammalian pyruvate dehydrogenase complex (× 200 000), and various interpretative models of the complex, consisting of twenty spheres arranged as a pentagonal dodecahedron, viewed down: *A*, a 2-fold axis; *B*, a 3-fold axis; and *C*, a 5-fold axis of symmetry. Reproduced by permission of Reed and Oliver[45] and Brookhaven Laboratories.

(vi) Orderly interactions between enzymes and substrates of the pyruvate dehydrogenase complex

As has already been stated, lipoic acid is covalently linked to an ε-amino group of a lysine residue of lipoyl reductase. The lipoyl group of lipoyl reductase participates in the reductive acetylation reaction, the acetyl transfer reaction, and the dihydrolipoate dehydrogenase reactions (reactions 2, 3 and 4). The reductive acetylation reaction (2) involves an interaction of the lipoyl group with the 1-hydroxy-ethylthiamine pyrophosphate of pyruvate dehydrogenase, while the acetyl transferase reaction involves an interaction of the lipoyl group with coenzyme A. It has been pointed out by Reed and co-workers that these interactions occur in a complex in which movement of the enzymes is restricted and in which intermediates do not appear to dissociate. Reed and co-workers have suggested that the attachment of lipoic acid to the ε-amino group of a lysine residue provides a flexible arm, about 14-Å long, for the reactive dithiolane ring of lipoic acid. This may permit a rotation of the lipoyl group between the enzymes of the complex (Fig. 5). The net charge on the lipoyl group during its cycle of transformations is 0, −1, and −2. Reed and co-workers have suggested further that this change in charge may pro-

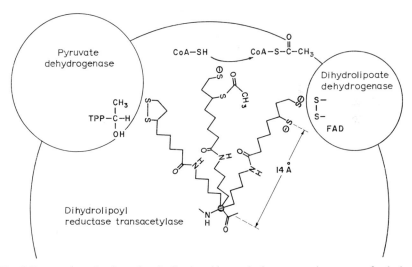

Fig. 5. Proposed mechanism whereby lipoic acid, attached to an ε-amino group of a lysine residue in lipoyl reductase–transacetylase, provides a flexible arm which ensures the orderly interaction between the enzymes of the pyruvate dehydrogenase complex and their various substrates. (Redrawn from Reed and Oliver[45])

vide for the driving force for moving the lipoyl group from one active site to the next[44,45].

(vii) *Occurrence of free forms of enzymes of the pyruvate dehydrogenase complex*

A survey of free and complexed forms of dihydrolipoate dehydrogenase in mitochondria has been reported. In the case of beef-heart mitochondria about 52% of the total dihydrolipoate dehydrogenase was found to be located in the pyruvate dehydrogenase complex, 23% in the α-ketoglutarate dehydrogenase complex, and 25% in the free form. The corresponding percentage location of the enzyme in beef liver mitochondria is 66, 6 and 28%, respectively. The authors used various mild procedures for breaking the mitochondria in order to avoid disrupting the dehydrogenase complexes themselves. If the dihydrolipoate dehydrogenase referred to as "free" is not in fact free, then this portion of the enzyme must be associated with a very labile complex of unknown nature[54]. No extramitochondrial lipoate dehydrogenase has been reported.

A careful survey for intra- or extramitochondrial free forms of the other enzymes of the pyruvate dehydrogenase complex does not so far appear to have been carried out, perhaps because assays of the partial reactions are technically difficult. One solution to this problem is to prepare antibodies to the isolated, pure enzymes separated from the complex, and to use these antibodies in search for the "free" enzymes[55].

In the case of bacterial pyruvate dehydrogenase, the component enzymes are produced in the correct proportions in which they are found in the complex. Since the component enzymes do not occur in the complex in simple one to one ratios, they must be synthesized at unequal rates[56].

(b) *Control of pyruvate oxidation*

(i) *Active and inactive forms of pyruvate dehydrogenase*

The activity of the pyruvate dehydrogenase complex isolated from beef kidney is regulated by phosphorylation and dephosphorylation. The highly purified complex is inactivated by incubation with ATP. The inactive preparation obtained in this manner is reactivated by incubation with magnesium ions. The phosphorylation and dephosphorylation are catalyzed by a kinase and a phosphatase which are associated with the pyruvate dehydrogenase complex[57].

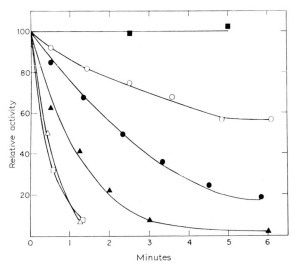

Fig. 6. Effect of incubating pyruvate dehydrogenase with ATP on pyruvate dehydrogenase activity. Incubation mixtures contained 20 mM potassium phosphate buffer, pH 7.0, 1 mM MgCl$_2$, 10 mM dithiothreitol, and pyruvate dehydrogenase (0.26 mg protein) in a total volume of 1.0 ml. The mixtures also contained the following amounts of ATP: ■, none; ○, 1 μM; ●, 5 μM; ▲, 10 μM; △, 100 μM; and □, 1 mM. The complete mixtures were incubated at 25°. At the indicated times 20-μl aliquots were withdrawn and pyruvate dehydrogenase activity was assayed by measuring the rate of production of NADH. (Reproduced from ref. 57, by permission of the authors and the Proceedings of the National Academy of Sciences.)

The effect of incubating the enzyme complex with ATP is shown in Fig. 6. The inactivation of the enzyme in the presence of 0.1 or 1mM ATP *plus* 1 mM Mg^{2+} is 90% complete in about one minute. The activity of enzyme complex inactivated in this manner is not restored by dilution, by dialysis, or by gel filtration.

The actual phosphorylation of the complex can be demonstrated using ^{32}P-labeled ATP. Radioactivity is incorporated from γ-labeled ATP, but not from α-labeled ATP. Various chemical treatments of the labeled protein suggest that the phosphoryl group is attached to a hydroxyl group on the enzyme.

Some preparations of phosphorylated pyruvate dehydrogenase complex were reactivated by incubation with Mg^{2+}, the optimum concentration being 10 mM. The material released was identified as orthophosphate by its solubility in isobutanol in the presence of molybdic acid. Other preparations underwent little reactivation in the presence of magnesium ions. This appears to be due to a lack in these preparations of a phosphatase. The latter was found to occur in protein fractions obtained in the later steps of the purification of the pyruvate dehydrogenase complex. When such fractions were added to the ATP-inactivated complex, restoration of activity was found to occur[57]. It follows that the phosphatase is associated relatively loosely with the pyruvate dehydrogenase complex.

Phosphorylation with ATP did not affect the acetyl transferase or dihydrolipoate dehydrogenase activities of the complex. The phosphorylated complex was resolved into lipoyl reductase–acetyl transferase, pyruvate decarboxylase, and dihydrolipoate dehydrogenase by Sepharose chromatography and salt fractionation. Essentially all of the protein-bound radioactivity was found in the pyruvate decarboxylase fraction. This enzyme contained about two moles of phosphate per mole of enzyme based on a molecular weight of 160 000.

The phosphorylation of pyruvate decarboxylase by pyruvate decarboxylase kinase, and the dephosphorylation of phosphorylated pyruvate decarboxylase by the corresponding phosphatase must both be under metabolic control. The data of Reed and co-workers[57] show that for optimum activity the phosphatase requires a magnesium ion concentration about ten times higher than the kinase. This suggests that the kinase and phosphatase activity may be regulated by the concentration of free magnesium ions. Reed and co-workers[57] have proposed that the free magnesium ion concentration is controlled in turn by the ratio of concentrations [ATP]/[ADP]. This interpretation fits certain observations, such as the reversal by uncouplers of oxidative phosphorylation of the inhibition of pyruvate oxidation brought about by fatty acids. However, as is shown below, a considerable number of variables change more or less at the same time, and it has not so far proven possible to identify definitively by metabolite assays the metabolites which serve as primary regulators of pyruvate dehydrogenase.

Control of activity by phosphorylation and dephosphorylation is well established in the case of glycogen phosphorylase[58] and glycogen synthetase[59]. In these cases the respective kinases and phosphatases are themselves under control. Thus phosphorylase b kinase is regulated by a cascade process involving various further enzymes, and cyclic AMP at or near the far end of the cascade. The active and inactive forms of pyruvate dehydrogenase were first reported[57] when this article was being written. If glycogen phosphorylase and glycogen synthetase constitute a relevant precedent, it is certain that

much remains to be uncovered about the phosphorylation and dephosphorylation of pyruvate dehydrogenase.

(ii) Control in the context of various metabolic pathways

Evidence which has been accumulated using various types of more or less
"intact" tissues indicates that pyruvate oxidation may be regulated by the
levels of acetyl-CoA and CoA, NADH and NAD, and ATP and ADP.
The controlling parameters may actually be the ratios of concentrations
[acetyl-CoA]/[CoA], [NADH]/[NAD] and [ATP]/[ADP]. These ratios all
change under conditions which cause a change in the rate of pyruvate
oxidation. So far, it has proven difficult to determine which of these changes,
if any, serve as primary controls.

Observations on a number of different tissues and tissue preparations
show that the oxidation of pyruvate is inhibited by fatty acids and *vice versa*.
Some of these systems have been studied in detail with the aim of understanding the control properties of pyruvate dehydrogenase and of the
metabolic system of which the enzyme complex is a part.

Observations with heart and other muscle. The oxidation of pyruvate by
perfused rat heart and by rat diaphragm is inhibited by fatty acids and
ketone bodies. Induction of diabetes leads to increased intracellular concentrations of fatty acids and ketone bodies, and is associated with a reduced
rate of pyruvate oxidation[60-62]. The two effects are clearly similar. Their
probable basis is the competitive inhibition of the pyruvate dehydrogenase
(reaction 5) by one of its products, namely acetyl-CoA[63]. The K_i for acetyl-
CoA is 12.5 μM while the K_m for CoA is 6.7 μM for the partially purified
enzyme from pigeon heart[63]. The intracellular level of acetyl-CoA is increased by fatty acids and ketone bodies, and in diabetes. A typical value for
acetyl-CoA in normal rat hearts perfused with glucose is 9 μM. Addition to
the perfusate of β-hydroxybutyrate, or acetate, or butyrate leads to levels of
about 85 μM. The level of acetyl-CoA in alloxan diabetic hearts is 71 μM[63].
These changes in concentration of acetyl-CoA indicate that inhibition of
reaction 5 by acetyl-CoA may be one of the control mechanisms responsible
for the inhibition of pyruvate oxidation. This assumes that the kinetic
parameters for pyruvate dehydrogenase in rat tissues are similar to those
reported for the pigeon heart enzyme.

Pyruvate dehydrogenase of *Escherichia coli* is inhibited by NADH[64-66].
In the case of the mammalian enzyme, the acetyl-CoA inhibition depends on

the presence of NADH, the 3-acetylpyridine analog of NADH being ineffective[67]. Whether NADH by itself is an inhibitor is not yet clear. The level of mitochondrial NADH increases upon initiation of fatty acid oxidation; the direction of this change is consistent with the regulation of pyruvate dehydrogenase by NADH.

Observations with liver preparations. In liver the main routes of acetyl-CoA production are the oxidation of pyruvate and the β-oxidation of fatty acids. The main routes of acetyl-CoA utilization are by the synthesis of citrate or acetoacetate. Control of acetyl-CoA metabolism thus involves a choice between alternate pathways in its synthesis, and between alternate pathways in its removal. This means ultimately that the rate at which each pathway operates must be regulated. The oxidation of pyruvate and the β-oxidation of fatty acids occur in the mitochondria, as does most of citrate and acetoacetate synthesis.

Another major route of pyruvate utilization in liver, and to a lesser extent in kidney, is that of gluconeogenesis[68,69]. Pyruvate enters this pathway through the pyruvate carboxylase reaction (11). The enzyme is activated by acetyl-CoA.

$$\text{Pyruvate} + \text{ATP} + CO_2 \xrightarrow{\text{acetyl-CoA}} \text{oxaloacetate} + \text{ADP} + P_i \quad (11)$$

A number of control mechanisms must operate to divert pyruvate from oxidation towards hexose synthesis. Oxidation of pyruvate is inhibited strongly by physiological concentrations of palmitate and palmityl carnitine[62,67,70,71]. On the other hand, gluconeogenesis is stimulated by fatty acid oxidation both *in vivo* and in homogenates[72-76]. As has already been mentioned, pyruvate dehydrogenase may be inhibited by acetyl-CoA, while pyruvate carboxylase is activated by this substance[77]. Thus an elevation in the level of acetyl-CoA is likely to contribute to the switch-over from pyruvate oxidation to pyruvate carboxylation. The concomitant lowering of the level of coenzyme A may also contribute to the reduced rate of pyruvate oxidation.

An experiment with mitochondria from liver of rat which demonstrates the effect of fatty acids on pyruvate oxidation is shown in Table I. In this experiment the citric acid cycle was blocked with fluorocitrate and malonate. The CO_2 output was therefore due only to pyruvate oxidation. Addition of

TABLE I

INHIBITION OF PYRUVATE OXIDATION BY PALMITYL CARNITINE

Rat-liver mitochondria (1.2 mg protein/ml), 5 mM pyruvate, 5 mM malate, 8 mM malonate, 10 μM fluorocitrate, 2 mM AMP, 2 mM MgCl$_2$, 1 mM EDTA, 80 mM KCl, 20 mM Tris–HCl, pH 7.2, temp. 37°. The rates shown have been calculated from the data of Nicholls et al.[71]. See also ref. 67.

Remarks	Oxygen uptake (natoms/mg/min)	CO$_2$ output (nmoles/mg/min)
None	57	59
Added 14 μM DL-palmityl carnitine	135	21
After oxidation of palmityl carnitine	79	54

palmityl carnitine increases the oxygen uptake and decreases the CO$_2$ output, the ratio of these two entities changes by a factor of 7. Once the palmityl carnitine has been consumed, oxygen uptake and CO$_2$ output return to their previous values, or nearly so.

The imposition of fatty acid oxidation on mitochondria which are oxidizing pyruvate leads to an increase in the ratio [acetyl-CoA]/[CoA][78]. The inhibition of pyruvate oxidation by fatty acids is prevented by dinitrophenol. The increase in the ratio [acetyl-CoA]/[CoA] is similarly prevented by dinitrophenol (Table II). It might be concluded that acetyl-CoA, or free CoA, or both exert a direct effect on pyruvate dehydrogenase. However, the addition of an uncoupling agent to mitochondria produces other changes in metabolic parameters, including a lowering of the ratios [ATP]/[ADP] and [NADH]/[NAD]. The experiment just described, while implicating [acetyl-CoA]/[CoA] as a controlling parameter, is not by itself conclusive.

TABLE II

COA AND ACETYL-COA IN RAT LIVER MITOCHONDRIA DURING THE OXIDATION OF PYRUVATE AND PALMITYL CARNITINE

Substrates	[CoA]	[acetyl-CoA]	[acetyl-CoA]
	(nmoles/mg protein)		[CoA]
Coupled oxidative phosphorylation			
Malate + pyruvate	0.39	0.08	0.20
Malate + pyruvate + palmityl carnitine	0.14	0.24	1.72
Uncoupled oxidative phosphorylation			
Malate + pyruvate	0.78	0.05	0.06
Malate + pyruvate + palmityl carnitine	0.35	0.10	0.29

Reproduced by permission of Garland et al.[67].

2. Citric acid cycle

(a) Introduction

The citric acid cycle is the final common pathway in the degradation of foodstuffs and cell constituents to carbon dioxide and water in most living organisms[79-82]. The bulk of the foodstuffs is digested to hexoses, amino acids, fatty acids, and glycerol. In the majority of cases these substances are then degraded to acetyl-coenzyme A. For example, hexoses are first converted to pyruvate and then to acetyl-coenzyme A, all fatty acids with an even number of carbon atoms are oxidized to acetyl-coenzyme A, and about one-half of the carbon skeletons of amino acids yield acetyl-coenzyme A. Some amino acids are degraded to one of the other members of the cycle. For example, glutamate, histidine, arginine, citrulline, ornithine, proline and hydroxyproline give rise to α-ketoglutarate; aspartate gives rise to oxaloacetate; isoleucine, valine, methionine, α-aminobutyric acid, propionic acid, and the three terminal carbon atoms of fatty acids with an uneven number of carbon atoms give rise to succinate; the benzene rings of tyrosine and phenylalanine give rise to fumarate[81-83]. These reactions are fully discussed

---

Fig. 7. The major reactions of the citric acid cycle. One turn of the cycle leads to the complete combustion of one molecule of acetic acid which enters the cycle as acetyl-coenzyme A. The dehydrogenase reactions lead to the formation of four pairs of $(H^+ + H^-)$. Three of these pairs are transferred to pyridine nucleotide coenzymes, in the isocitrate, α-ketoglutarate and malate dehydrogenase reactions; the fourth pair is transferred to flavin–adenine dinucleotide in the succinate dehydrogenase reaction. The other end products are two molecules of CO_2. The elements of water are added and eliminated at several stages. Some or all of the hydrogen removed in the dehydrogenase reactions reacts with molecular oxygen through the respiratory chain to form water. Most of the reactions have been shown to be reversible *in vitro*. For simplicity, reversibility is not indicated in the diagram. Although the formulas show the free acids, the compounds participate in the cycle in the form of their anions, and they are named as such. The carbon atoms fed into the cycle in the form of acetyl-coenzyme A are shown in heavy outline, and their fate is traced to the point where they reach succinate. This pair of carbon atoms remains in the compounds of the cycle during their first turn around the cycle. The reactions shown are catalyzed by the following enzymes: a, citrate synthase (condensing enzyme); b_1 and b_2, aconitase; c, isocitrate dehydrogenase; d, α-ketoglutarate dehydrogenase; e, succinyl-CoA synthetase (succinate thiokinase); f, succinate dehydrogenase; g, fumarase; h, malate dehydrogenase. Some qualifying remarks: (*1*) *cis*-Aconitate is not an obligatory, free intermediate in the aconitase reaction. (*2*) Oxalosuccinate may occur as an enzyme-bound intermediate in the isocitrate dehydrogenase reaction. (*3*) In brain the α-ketoglutarate dehydrogenase reaction can be circumvented by the γ-aminobutyrate pathway. (*4*) Succinate can also be derived from succinyl-coenzyme A by the reactions catalyzed by succinyl-CoA–acetoacetate-CoA transferase and by succinyl-CoA deacylase.

in other parts of this series. The processes enumerated above apply to animal tissues as well as microorganisms. The latter possess additional reactions which are capable of converting many other substances to intermediates of the cycle.

An outline of the major reactions of the citric acid cycle is shown in Fig. 7. One complete turn of the cycle results in the combustion of one molecule of

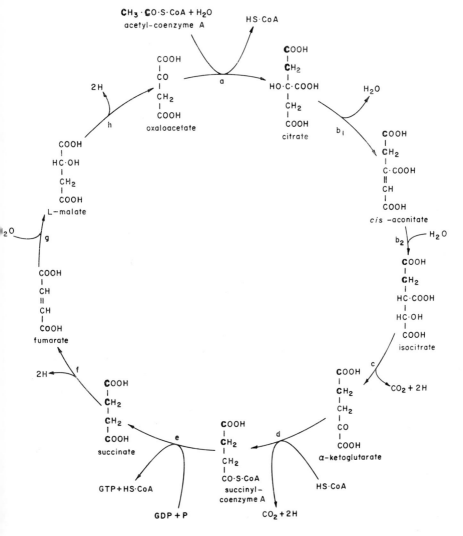

acetic acid to carbon dioxide and water. The stoichiometry of this process is as follows:

$$CH_3 \cdot COOH + 2H_2O \rightarrow 2CO_2 + 8[H] \qquad (12)$$
$$8[H] + 2O_2 \rightarrow 4H_2O \qquad (13)$$

$$\text{Sum: } CH_3 \cdot COOH + 2O_2 \rightarrow 2CO_2 + 2H_2O \qquad (14)$$

This summary is an oversimplification which ignores that acetic acid reacts in the form of acetyl-coenzyme A, and that charged molecules are involved in the process as a whole.

Carbon dioxide arises directly as a result of the isocitrate and α-ketoglutarate dehydrogenase reactions. Four pairs of hydrogen atoms are removed by four different oxidative reactions of the cycle, which are catalyzed by isocitrate, α-ketoglutarate, succinate and malate dehydrogenases. Each pair of hydrogen atoms is transferred to a coenzyme. Mammalian tissues possess two main types of isocitrate dehydrogenases which differ by being NAD- or NADP-specific. α-Ketoglutarate and malate dehydrogenases are NAD-specific, and succinate dehydrogenase is FAD-specific. When the cycle serves in its function of supplying energy for the resynthesis of ATP from ADP, the hydrogen atoms are transferred to the enzymes of the electron-transport chain. In the course of this transfer they become dissociated into protons and electrons (Eqn. 15). The electrons pass through the enzymes of the electron-transport (or cytochrome) chain and are ultimately used to reduce oxygen. The net result is the combination of hydrogen and oxygen to form water:

$$4[H] \rightarrow 4H^+ + 4e \qquad (15)$$
$$O_2 + 4e \rightarrow 2O^{2-} \qquad (16)$$
$$4H^+ + 2O^{2-} \rightarrow 2H_2O \qquad (17)$$

$$\text{Sum: } 4[H] + O_2 \rightarrow 2H_2O \qquad (18)$$

The passage of the electrons from reduced coenzymes through the electron-transport chain to oxygen is obligatorily linked to the synthesis of ATP from ADP and orthophosphate. In other words, respiration is coupled to phosphorylation.

The tightness of the coupling of oxidative phosphorylation, that is to say the efficiency of the conversion of energy into ATP, may be one of the factors which determines whether excess caloric intake is wasted to some extent, or is stored. Energy is stored in two forms: carbohydrate and fat. The size of the carbohydrate stores is limited; the size of the fat stores is virtually unlimited.

A small difference in the efficiency of energy conversion may, over a period of time, make a large difference in the amount of fat stored.

All of the enzymes of the citric acid cycle have been highly purified[84]. The stereochemistry of each reaction of the cycle has been established with respect to all carbon and hydrogen atoms. A detailed account of the properties of the enzymes and of the stereochemical interrelations has been given in a recent article[82] and will not be repeated here.

(b) Intracellular compartmentation of enzymes of the citric acid cycle

Animal cells generally contain well-defined nuclei, mitochondria, rough-surfaced and smooth-surfaced endoplasmic reticulum, and, in some cases, lysozomes and related particles. Electron micrographs of typical mitochondria from liver and muscle of rat are shown in Fig. 8 A and B. A diagram of an idealized mitochondrion is shown in Fig. 8 C. These pictures are intended to assist the reader in the discussions of compartmentation which follow. Details of mitochondrial ultrastructure have been reviewed elsewhere[85-90]. In this section intracellular compartmentation is considered from two points of view: compartmentation of enzymes and of metabolites.

Green and co-workers[91] first demonstrated that rabbit kidney particles ("cyclophorase") can completely oxidize pyruvate and most of the intermediates of the citric acid cycle. Shortly afterwards it was shown that these oxidative reactions are associated with the mitochondrial fraction of rat liver. Little of these reactions was found in nuclear and microsomal fractions[92,93]. It soon became accepted that mitochondria contain all the enzymes of the citric acid cycle[94,95], but these studies left open the question of whether the enzymes of the citric acid cycle occur *only* in the mitochondria[96,97]. Originally it was thought that citric acid cycle enzymes which were found in the extramitochondrial fractions might be artifacts derived from the mitochondria during the breakage of the cell. This was shown not to be the case by the use of "marker" enzymes[98,99]. The choice of marker enzymes depends somewhat on the tissue. For example in the case of liver, cytochrome oxidase can serve as an "insoluble" mitochondrial marker enzyme, and glutamate dehydrogenase can serve as a soluble, mitochondrial enzyme, that is an enzyme which readily passes into solution when the mitochondrial membranes are damaged either mechanically, chemically, or enzymatically. If an enzyme is found in the particle-free supernatant obtained by centrifuging a homogenate, and if the soluble, mitochondrial marker enzyme is

TABLE III

INTRACELLULAR DISTRIBUTION OF CITRIC ACID CYCLE AND ANCILLARY ENZYMES IN MAMMALIAN TISSUES

Unless otherwise indicated the distribution studies refer to rat organs.

Enzymes	Organ	Location of activity[a]		References
		Mitochondria	Non-particulate cytoplasm	
A. Citric acid cycle enzymes				
Citrate synthase	Heart	95	5	101–103
Aconitase	Brain, liver	75–85	20–35	105–109
Isocitrate dehydrogenase				
NAP-specific	Heart, brain	100	0	108, 110–114, 179
NADP-specific[b]	Liver	15	85	103, 106, 112, 114–122
	Brain	55	45	179
α-Ketoglutarate dehydrogenase complex[c]	Heart	20–55	—	129, 130
Succinyl-CoA synthetase	Liver, kidney	100	0	131
Succinyl-CoA–aceto-acetate-CoA transferase[d]	Kidney	95	5	131
	Heart	41	54	131
Succinyl-CoA hydrolase[e]	Liver	70	30	131
	Kidney	65	35	
Succinate dehydrogenase	Heart, liver	100	0	132, 133, but see 136, 137
Fumarase	Brain	70	30	106, 107, 137, 140, 141
	Liver	50	50	
Malate dehydrogenase[f]	Various	~45	~55	142–147
B. Some major ancillary enzymes				
Pyruvate dehydrogenase complex[g]	Various	100	0	See page 12
Citrate cleavage enzyme	Liver[h]	0	100	104
Glutamate dehydrogenase	Liver	100	0	171
Aspartate aminotransferase[f]	Liver / Kidney	~50	~50	172–177

| Enzymes | Organ | Location of activity[a] | | References |
		Mitochondria	Non-particulate cytoplasm	
Malic enzyme	Liver[h]	<9	90–100	178
	Brain	75	25	179
	Adipose tissue	2	98	188
Pyruvate carboxylase	Liver (rat)	76–91	24–29	183–185, 187
	Liver (rat)	100	0	186
	Liver (chicken)	100	0	182
	Brain	100	0	186
	Adipose tissue	57–68	43–32	185, 188
	Lactating mammary gland (rat)	80	20	189
	(rabbit)	0	100	189
Phosphoenolpyruvate carboxykinase	Liver, depending on species[i]	0–100	100–0	187, 190, 191, see Table IV
	Adipose tissue	12	88	194

[a] Expressed as percent of total activity to nearest 5%.

[b] The intra- and extramitochondrial enzymes differ from each other. The percentage distribution is based on the sum of the activities of the two NADP-specific enzymes. Some of the activity attributed to the mitochondria actually may be located in the peroxizomes (see text). For a more detailed account of intracellular distribution studies of isocitrate dehydrogenases the reader is referred to ref. 127.

[c] Assayed as α-ketoglutarate oxidase activity. A poor recovery of total activity was obtained using mitochondria in the absence of other cell components.

[d] Activity absent or extremely low in liver.

[e] Values are approximate because rates proportional to protein concentration were not obtained.

[f] The intra- and extramitochondrial enzymes differ from each other. The percentage distribution is based on the sum of the activities of the two enzymes.

[g] Assayed as pyruvate oxidase activity. No survey of the corresponding dehydrogenase activity appears to have been made. The general opinion to be found in the literature is that pyruvate dehydrogenase is exclusively intramitochondrial.

[h] This distribution study was performed on pigeon liver.

[i] See Table IV.

absent from the same preparation, then it is assumed that the enzyme in question occurs extramitochondrially.

More sophisticated criteria have come into use in recent years, and more subtle distinctions are beginning to be made for intramitochondrial enzymes than the simple one of "soluble" and "insoluble"[86]. Among the most efficient methods is the examination of the integrity of the isolated mitochondria or other particles by electron microscopy.

A brief overview is given below of the intracellular compartmentation of the individual enzymes of the citric acid cycle, as well as of some ancillary enzymes of the cycle (Table III). In much of this work the criteria of marker enzymes and electron microscopy were not used. Nevertheless, it is now clear that although some of the enzymes of the citric acid cycle are largely or exclusively confined to the mitochondria[97,100], others occur partially and in some cases predominantly in the cytoplasm.

(i) Citrate synthase and ATP:citrate lyase

Citrate synthase occurs exclusively, or almost exclusively, in the mitochondria[101-103]. While the citrate synthase reaction (19) is readily reversible

$$\text{Acetyl-CoA} + \text{oxaloacetate} + H_2O \leftrightarrow \text{citrate} + \text{CoA} \qquad (19)$$

in vitro, it is unlikely that the reverse reaction catalyzed by this enzyme is of importance *in vivo*. In higher animals, the direct conversion of citrate to acetyl-CoA and oxaloacetate is catalyzed by ATP:citrate lyase (citrate cleavage enzyme) (reaction 20). In contrast to citrate synthase, citrate cleavage enzyme is found largely in the non-particulate, extramitochondrial space of the cell[104].

$$\text{Citrate} + \text{CoA} + \text{ATP} \rightarrow$$
$$\text{acetyl-CoA} + \text{oxaloacetate} + \text{ADP} + \text{orthophosphate} \qquad (20)$$

(ii) Aconitase

The enzyme has been reported to occur both intra- and extramitochondrially[105-109], the exact distribution depending on the organ and

$$\text{Citrate} \leftrightarrow \text{cis-aconitate} + H_2O \leftrightarrow \text{isocitrate} \qquad (21)$$

species. The intra- and extramitochondrial aconitases have not been characterized sufficiently to make possible a decision whether they differ from one another or are identical.

(*iii*) *Isocitrate dehydrogenases*

Higher animals possess both NAD- and NADP-specific enzymes which differ in their intracellular distribution. The NAD-specific enzyme is found

$$\text{Isocitrate} + \text{NAD}^+ \leftrightarrow \alpha\text{-ketoglutarate} + CO_2 + \text{NADH} + H^+ \quad (22a)$$

$$\text{Isocitrate} + \text{NADP}^+ \leftrightarrow \alpha\text{-ketoglutarate} + CO_2 + \text{NADPH} + H^+ \quad (22b)$$

only in mitochondria[108,110-114]. NADP-specific enzymes occur both in the particulate fractions and in the particle-free cytoplasm[103,106,112,114-119]. For example, in rat liver about 15% of the total NADP-specific enzyme activity occurs in the mitochondria and the remainder in the cytoplasm[118,120-122]. The intra- and extramitochondrial, NADP-specific isocitrate dehydrogenases differ from each other in electrophoretic mobility and in immunological properties[113,122].

Recent work shows that some of the activity previously attributed to mitochondria may in fact be associated with peroxisomes, particles which belong to the general category of lysozomes. The peroxisomes of *Tetrahymena pyriformis* resemble the peroxisomes of mammalian liver and kidney in their enzymatic composition and in their sedimentation properties[123-125]. In addition it has been shown that in *T.pyriformis* two key enzymes of the glyoxylate cycle, isocitrate lyase and malate synthase, are associated with special particles[126]. De Duve and co-workers demonstrated that these particles are peroxisomes[125]. Most of particle-associated enzymes of the citric acid cycle are found exclusively in the mitochondrial fraction and not in the peroxisomes. However in the case of *T.pyriformis*, 40% of the NADP specific isocitrate dehydrogenase is associated with the peroxisomes, 5% with the mitochondria, and the remainder with the non-particulate fraction[125].

Isocitrate lyase and malate synthase do not occur in mammalian tissues; nevertheless, it has been found that peroxisomes prepared from rat liver also contain small amounts of NADP-specific isocitrate dehydrogenase[127]. In the case of endosperm of the germinating castor bean, all the enzymes of the glyoxylate cycle have been reported to occur in a particle which can be separated from mitochondria by density gradient centrifugation. This particle, which is similar in a number of respects to the peroxisome, has been referred to as glyoxysome[128]. At present it is difficult to assess the metabolic significance of the NADP-specific isocitrate dehydrogenase in peroxisomes.

It has been suggested that since the reaction catalyzed by the enzyme is reversible, it may provide an alternate source of isocitrate for the glyoxylate cycle at the expense of α-ketoglutarate and its amino acid precursors. This hypothesis seems reasonable in the case of *T.pyriformis*, but it leaves open the function of isocitrate dehydrogenase in mammalian peroxisomes.

(iv) α-Ketoglutarate dehydrogenase complex

Very little work has been done concerning the intracellular distribution of the component enzymes of this complex. α-Ketoglutarate oxidase activity is confined to the mitochondria[129,130]. In mammalian systems, assays of

$$\alpha\text{-Ketoglutarate} + NAD^+ + CoA \leftrightarrow \text{succinyl-CoA} + CO_2 + NADH + H^+ \quad (23)$$

oxidase activity are really measures of cytochrome oxidase, an enzyme generally agreed to be confined to the inner membrane of mitochondria. No survey of the distribution of α-ketoglutarate dehydrogenase appears to have been made. Although the general opinion to be found in the literature is that this enzyme is exclusively intramitochondrial, it is pertinent that in one of the α-ketoglutarate oxidase studies mentioned above[129], only 20% of the total activity was recovered in the mitochondrial fraction. The possibility therefore exists that some of the components of the α-ketoglutarate dehydrogenase complex exist in the extramitochondrial fraction of the mammalian cell.

(v) Succinate thiokinase, succinyl-CoA–acetoacetate-CoA transferase and succinyl-CoA hydrolase

Succinyl-CoA formed in the α-ketoglutarate dehydrogenase reaction can be converted to succinate in three different reactions:

$$\text{Succinyl-CoA} + GDP + P_i \leftrightarrow \text{succinate} + GTP + CoA \quad (24)$$

$$\text{Succinyl-CoA} + \text{acetoacetate} \leftrightarrow \text{succinate} + \text{acetoacetyl-CoA} \quad (25)$$

$$\text{Succinyl-CoA} + H_2O \leftrightarrow \text{succinate} + CoA \quad (26)$$

In liver, the succinyl-CoA synthetase (succinate thiokinase) reaction (24) can account for about 80% of the total capacity to convert succinyl-CoA to succinate. The hydrolase reaction (26) can account for as much as 20% of the total capacity of liver, while the succinyl-CoA–acetoacetate-CoA transferase reaction (25) can account for less than one percent[131].

In heart, leg muscle, and kidney, succinyl-CoA hydrolase activity can account for less than 3% of the total capacity to convert succinyl-CoA to succinate. In these three tissues succinyl-CoA–acetoacetate-CoA transferase activity is considerably greater than succinate thiokinase.

Concerning the intracellular distribution of these enzymes, succinyl-CoA synthetase is predominantly intramitochondrial. Succinyl-CoA–acetoacetate-CoA transferase is mainly intramitochondrial in kidney and leg muscle, but it appears to be approximately evenly distributed between the intra- and extramitochondrial fractions of heart homogenates. Succinyl-CoA hydrolase is somewhat more concentrated in the mitochondria than in the cytoplasm[131]. It seems likely that the measurements of succinyl-CoA hydrolase activity reflect various thioesterase activities rather than a specific succinyl-CoA deacylase.

(vi) Succinate dehydrogenase

Relatively few studies have been reported of the intracellular distribution of succinate dehydrogenase, probably because it has long been considered an example of an insoluble, mitochondrial enzyme[132,133]. However, it should be

$$\text{Succinate} + 2 \text{ cyt. } b \text{ (Fe}^{3+}) \leftrightarrow \text{fumarate} + 2 \text{ cyt. } b \text{ (Fe}^{2+}) + 2\text{H}^+ \quad (27)$$

pointed out that all of the early work involved either an oxidase assay, which is really a measure of the distribution of cytochrome oxidase, or an assay with a dye-acceptor which required some mitochondrial component of the respiratory chain[97,134]. Assays of succinate dehydrogenase with ferricyanide or phenazinemethosulfate[135] do not depend on components of the respiratory chain. They thus provide a measure of the activity of succinate dehydrogenase itself. However, mammalian mitochondria possess permeability barriers to electron acceptors of this type[135], which means that the insides of the mitochondria must be exposed by mechanical or other damage before the full activity of the enzyme can be assessed. Measurements of succinate dehydrogenase activity before and after breaking the mitochondrial permeability barrier to direct electron acceptors do not appear to have been made so far. Nevertheless, there is some indication that a portion of the enzyme may occur outside the mitochondria in some circumstances[136,137].

On sonicating rat-liver mitochondria, about 8% of the total succinate dehydrogenase activity present in the mitochondria is released into the soluble fraction at the same rapid rate as isocitrate, malate, and sarcosine dehydrogenases. Freezing and thawing of mitochondria results in the rapid release of about 4% of the succinate dehydrogenase[109]. The remaining 92–96% of the succinate dehydrogenase activity is not released by this type of treatment. This "insoluble" enzyme can be brought into solution by treatment with organic solvents such as butanol[138,139].

(vii) Fumarase

Distribution studies show that fumarase occurs both in the intra- and the extramitochondrial space of the cell.

$$\text{Fumarate} + H_2O \leftrightarrow \text{L-malate} \qquad (28)$$

In brain about two-thirds of the enzyme is found in the mitochondria, with the remainder in the high-speed supernatant fraction. In liver the activity of fumarase is about evenly divided between these compartments[106,107,137, 140,141]. The intra- and extramitochondrial fumarases have not been characterized sufficiently to make possible a decision whether they differ from one another or are identical. Intramitochondrial fumarase is a non-particulate enzyme, its rate of release from the mitochondria being the same as that of isocitrate, malate and sarcosine dehydrogenases, as well as aconitase[109].

(viii) Malate dehydrogenases

All tissues of higher animals which have been examined so far contain both intra- and extramitochondrial malate dehydrogenases. The activity is about equally divided between these two compartments[142–147]. Both types of enzyme have been isolated in highly purified form from a number of

$$\text{L-Malate} + NAD^+ \leftrightarrow \text{oxaloacetate} + NADH + H^+ \qquad (29)$$

sources[148–154]. The intra- and extramitochondrial enzymes are different proteins. This is evident from differences in molecular weight, electrophoretic mobility, and amino acid composition[147,155–159]. Other differences between the two types of malate dehydrogenase abound, including differences in stability, chromatographic behavior, thiol group content, and coenzyme binding[86]. It was reported that the intramitochondrial enzyme from a number of species lacks tryptophan[157,159–161], but more recent work shows that this finding was probably incorrect[162].

Plants[163] and Neurospora crassa[164] also possess different intra- and extramitochondrial malate dehydrogenases. The enzyme from Bacillus subtilis, *Escherichia coli*, and *Pseudomonas acidovansis* is NAD-specific[154, 165-168]. The readiness with which the enzyme from *E. coli* passes into solution upon cell breakage suggests that the enzyme occurs in the soluble fraction of the cell. Malate dehydrogenase from *Acetobacter xylinum* and *Pseudomonas ovalis* Chester is FAD-linked. Ultrasonic disruption of cells containing this enzyme, followed by centrifugation, shows that more than 90% of the enzyme activity is particulate[169,170].

(c) Compartmentation of some enzymes ancillary to the citric acid cycle

A number of enzymes catalyze reactions that lead to and from compounds of the citric acid cycle. The intracellular distribution of some of the more important of these will now be considered.

(i) Pyruvate dehydrogenase complex

In higher animals the pyruvate dehydrogenase complex appears to occur exclusively in the mitochondria. As has already been mentioned (p. 12), an intracellular distribution study of the free forms of the constituent enzymes of the complex has not so far been reported.

(ii) ATP:citrate lyase (citrate cleavage enzyme)

The reaction catalyzed by this enzyme is shown in Eqn. 20. An intracellular distribution study has shown it to occur largely in the cytoplasm[104].

(iii) Glutamate dehydrogenase

This enzyme is found exclusively in mitochondria of liver[171], and it is commonly used as a mitochondrial marker enzyme in studies of intracellular enzyme distribution in liver.

$$\alpha\text{-Ketoglutarate} + NH_4^+ + NADH (NADPH) \leftrightarrow$$
$$\text{glutamate} + NAD^+ (NADP^+) \quad (30)$$

(iv) Aspartate aminotransferase

The enzyme occurs in all tissues of higher animals in the form of intra- and extramitochondrial isozymes[172-175]. The total activity is about equally

$$\text{Aspartate} + \alpha\text{-ketoglutarate} \leftrightarrow \text{oxaloacetate} + \text{glutamate} \quad (31)$$

divided between mitochondria and cytoplasm of liver, kidney, and muscle[176,177].

References p. 49

(v) Malic enzyme

The enzyme found in pigeon liver occurs almost completely in the non-particulate cytoplasm[178].

$$Malate + NADP^+ \leftrightarrow pyruvate + CO_2 + NADPH + H^+ \qquad (32)$$

Rat brain possesses about the same level of malic enzyme as rat liver, namely about 0.8 μmole of NADPH formed per g per min[179,180]. In contrast to liver, about 75% of the brain enzyme is found in the mitochondrial fraction[179]. The intra- and extramitochondrial brain enzymes and the liver enzyme possess similar kinetic properties[179,180]. Moreover, the brain and liver enzymes of mouse appear to be electrophoretically similar, although malic enzyme from heart mitochondria is different[181].

(vi) Pyruvate carboxylase

In chicken liver the activity of pyruvate carboxylase is largely confined to the mitochondria. Some activity is found in the homogenate fraction which sediments more rapidly than mitochondria and which contains nuclei and cell debris. Whether this activity is due to mitochondria trapped in the heavier fraction was not determined[182].

$$Pyruvate + ATP + CO_2 \xrightarrow{\text{acetyl-CoA}} oxaloacetate + ADP + P_i \qquad (11)$$

In liver of rat, 10–25% of the pyruvate carboxylase activity occurs in the non-particulate cytoplasm[183–185]. This finding is somewhat controversial since a recent paper reports that even in rat liver all but a trace of the activity occurs in the mitochondria[186].

Pyruvate carboxylase is present in brain of rat, although in relatively small amounts (0.2 μmole/g brain/min at 25°, ref. 179, compared to about 5 μmoles/g liver/min at 25°, ref. 187). The brain enzyme occurs entirely in the mitochondria[179].

In adipose tissue of rat about one-third of the activity is cytoplasmic[185,188]. In lactating mammary gland of rat one-fifth of the activity is cytoplasmic, but in lactating mammary gland of rabbit all of the activity is found in the mitochondria[189].

(vii) Phosphoenolpyruvate carboxykinase

The intracellular distribution of phosphoenolpyruvate carboxykinase in liver shows considerable species variation[187,190,191]. In mouse and hamster liver the enzyme is confined to the extramitochondrial, soluble fraction,

$$\text{Oxaloacetate} + GTP \rightarrow \text{phosphoenolpyruvate} + GDP + CO_2 \qquad (33)$$

while in rabbit and pigeon it is confined to the particulate fractions. Rat and guinea pig liver possess an intermediate distribution of the enzyme (Table IV). A search for possible differences between the intra- and extramitochondrial enzymes showed them to be kinetically very similar[187,192]. On the other hand, the intra- and extramitochondrial enzymes prepared from rat liver differ immunologically[193].

In adipose tissue about 12% of the activity of the enzyme is intramitochondrial, while the rest is found in the cytoplasm[194].

TABLE IV

INTRACELLULAR DISTRIBUTION OF PHOSPHOENOLPYRUVATE CARBOXYKINASE
ACTIVITY IN LIVER OF VARIOUS SPECIES

Total activities are expressed as μmoles of phosphoenolpyruvate formed per g of liver per min. Relative activities are expressed as percent of total activity. The particulate fractions were frozen and thawed eight times before assay. (From Nordlie and Lardy[190]). Note that the activity in pigeon liver is also confined to the particulate fraction[191].

	Mouse	Hamster	Rat	Guinea pig	Rabbit
Total activity[a]	3.3	2.1	9.5	36.6	5.9
Relative activity					
Non-particulate	100	100	83	33	c
Microsomes	c	c	4	c	c
Mitochondria	c	c	4	45	58
Nuclei[b]	c	c	9	22	42

a Sum of separate activities.
b Includes nuclei plus cellular debris.
c Activity undetectable.

(d) *Permeability of mitochondria to substrates of the citric acid cycle*

Mitochondria are relatively impermeable to most of the small molecules which occur in the cell. For example, Lehninger showed in 1951 that carefully isolated mitochondria do not oxidize externally added NADH[195]. Subsequently it was shown that intra- and extramitochondrial pyridine nucleotides do not equilibrate or exchange with each other *in vivo*, at least not at a rate which is significant in terms of the respiratory rate[196]. The permeability of mitochondria and other organelles to both anions and cations has been investigated extensively in recent years. This section is confined to a consideration of the permeability of mitochondria to citric acid cycle anions and closely related substances. A number of review articles and a book have been devoted largely to this topic[197–199].

The permeability properties of mitochondria towards compounds of the citric acid cycle, as well as towards mono- and dinucleotides and orthophosphate, reside in the inner mitochondrial membrane[86,198]. The soluble mitochondrial enzymes of the citric acid cycle and of related reactions, are localized in the matrix space of the mitochondria. The matrix space is surrounded by the inner mitochondrial membrane and is penetrated by the cristae (Fig. 8). The insoluble mitochondrial enzymes of the cycle, succinate dehydrogenase and the α-ketoacid dehydrogenases, are localized in or on the cristae and inner membrane[198,200]. It follows that for a substrate of the citric acid cycle to react with one of the mitochondrial citric acid cycle enzymes it must first of all penetrate into or through the inner membrane or cristae. "Insoluble" enzymes such as succinate dehydrogenase, which are located in the inner membrane, are only accessible to their substrates from the matrix side of the membrane[198].

Studies of the permeability properties of isolated mitochondria show that the inner mitochondrial membrane must contain a number of specific permeases or transporting enzymes which require activators before they function. In the absence of such activators, the inner mitochondrial membrane is relatively impermeable to most small molecules of physiological interest[198, 199].

Three techniques have been employed to study the penetration of the inner mitochondrial membrane by metabolites[198]. The first technique is based on a comparison of the penetration of three substances: ³H-labeled water, ¹⁴C-labeled sucrose, and the compound under study. Water and sucrose penetrate the space between the outer and inner membrane and probably the intracristal space. Water also penetrates the matrix space, where the soluble enzymes of the citric acid cycle are located. Sucrose does not penetrate this space unless the mitochondria are disrupted. The labeled water and sucrose are added first. After an equilibration period the substrate to be studied is added. The mitochondria are then centrifuged down at suitable intervals and the concentration of the substrate is measured in the supernatant and in the pellet. Experiments of this type showed that citrate or α-ketoglutarate penetrate only the space in the mitochondria which is accessible to sucrose, that is to say they do not penetrate the matrix space. In the presence of malate, both citrate and α-ketoglutarate penetrate all of the space available to the labeled water, that is to say they penetrate the matrix space as well as the space between the inner and outer membranes.

In order for this first technique to be applied successfully, the mitochondria must be at least partially depleted of endogenous substrates such as malate,

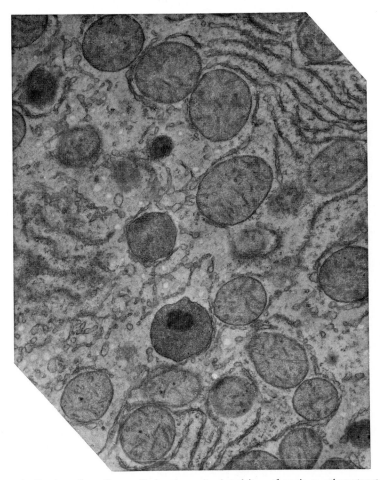

Fig. 8 A. Section of rat liver cell showing mitochondria and various other structures. Palade's fixative, embedded in Epon (× 40000).

References p. 49

and metabolism of the substrate being tested must be prevented after it enters the mitochondria. Inhibitors of substrate-level metabolism, such as fluorocitrate and arsenite, and of the respiratory chain, such as rotenone and antimycin, are suitable for this purpose. Another practical point is that penetration by an anion must be accompanied either by penetration of cations of equivalent charge or by exchange with another anion of equivalent charge. In practice it is simplest to provide a cation which can readily penetrate the mitochondrial membrane without being involved in energy-linked transport phenomena. Ammonium or methyl ammonium ions are suitable for this purpose. The inner mitochondrial membrane is normally almost impermeable to alkali metal cations; in the absence of energy metabolism, anions fail to penetrate when sodium or potassium ions are substituted for ammonium ions.

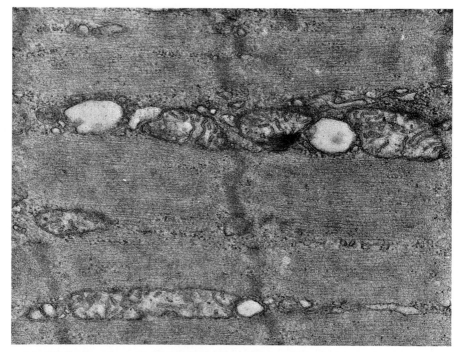

Fig. 8 B. Section of rat striated muscle showing mitochondria and various other structures. Palade's fixative, embedded in Araldite ($\times$ 59 000). The electron micrographs were kindly provided by Dr. Donald F. Parsons.

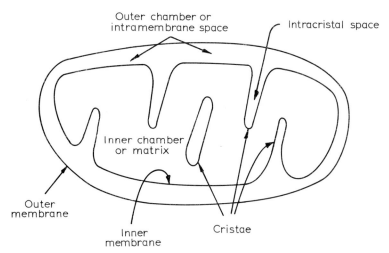

Fig. 8 C. Idealized section through a liver mitochondrion. The inner and outer membranes are about 55 Å thick. The intracristal space is shown to be in direct communication with the intramembrane space.

The second technique is based on measuring the osmotic behavior of mitochondria. This depends on the properties of the inner membrane. Chappell has discussed three variations of the technique[198]. In the first of these it is determined whether mitochondria swell in iso-osmotic solutions of the ammonium salts of the anion being studied. If the mitochondria swell rapidly, this is evidence that the anions penetrate readily. Results obtained using this approach are summarized in Table V[197,201]. It was found that of the common inorganic anions tested, only phosphate and arsenate readily penetrate liver mitochondria[201]. The technique served to show that the inner membrane of liver mitochondria possesses specific permeability properties with respect to di- and tricarboxylic acids of the citric acid cycle, and that the permeability to such compounds is subject to activation by orthophosphate and malate[197].

    In the second variation of the osmotic approach, the mitochondria are suspended in different concentrations of the ammonium salts of the anions. If the anion readily penetrates the mitochondria, there is an adjustment of osmotic pressure without change in volume. If the anion does *not* penetrate the inner mitochondrial membrane, there is an adjustment of osmotic pressure by a change in the mitochondrial volume. This technique was used to demonstrate that mitochondria behave as osmometers in ammonuim fumarate but not in ammonium succinate[197,198]. In other words the mitochondria are freely permeable to succinate but not to fumarate. Similarly, mitochondria were shown to behave as osmometers in the presence of ammonium citrate alone, but not when malate and phosphate were also present in addition to ammonium citrate.

In the third variation of the osmotic approach, small amounts of a concentrated solution of the ammonium salt of an anion are added to a suspension of mitochondria in an isotonic solution of ammonium chloride. When this is done the mitochondria contract initially to compensate for the sudden increase in the osmotic pressure of the medium. If the anion added can enter the mitochondria, the initial contraction is followed by swelling because the concentration of the anion becomes equalized on both sides of the inner membrane. If the anion cannot penetrate the inner membrane, the initial contraction is not followed by swelling.

Swelling and shrinking of mitochondria is most simply followed by measuring changes in light-scattering. In the first of the techniques described above, metabolism of the compound under study is deliberately prevented. In the second technique very high concentrations of the ammonium salt of the anion must be used in order to demonstrate the desired effects. It may be objected that both sets of conditions are unphysiological.

The third technique attempts to meet this objection. It involves measuring the changes in the redox state of intramitochondrial pyridine nucleotides, and it is thus limited to a study of *substrate* anions. This technique depends on the observation that the soluble, mitochondrial enzymes of the citric acid cycle are located in the matrix, and that the insoluble mitochondrial enzymes of the cycle are accessible from the inner side of the inner membrane only. Changes in the levels of reduced pyridine nucleotides can be measured by double-beam spectrophotometry, which automatically corrects for changes in light-scattering, or by fluorimetry. By this means it was shown, for example, that externally added isocitrate does not react in the intramitochondrial isocitrate dehydrogenase reaction, and externally added citrate does not react in the intramitochondrial aconitase reaction, unless another substance is added which facilitates the transfer of the tricarboxylic acids across the inner mitochondrial membrane[202-204]. As is discussed below, the facilitating or activating function is best served by L-malate. Controls show that L-malate does not affect the kinetics of isocitrate dehydrogenase and aconitase, and malate does not appear to exert any other activating effect.

Results obtained using the techniques just discussed have led to the conclusion that anions enter the mitochondrial matrix by exchange diffusion which is catalyzed by various permeases[197]. This type of entry does not require an energy supply, such as ATP or intermediates of oxidative phosphorylation, since the anions which penetrate into the mitochondrial matrix (see Table V) do so in the absence of respiration and the operation of of citric acid cycle.

The term *permease* is used to designate an enzyme or enzyme system located in a membrane which permits passage of certain specific substances across that membrane. A permease may be subject to regulation, that is, it may be activated or inhibited. A number of terms have been used in place of *permease*, including carrier system, transporting system, transporter, port and antiport, porter, translocase, and others. At present, none of these terms seems to be any improvement over the term permease, which implies an

TABLE V

ENTRY OF MITOCHONDRIAL MATRIX SPACE BY AMMONIUM SALTS OF VARIOUS ANIONS[a]

Enter without additions	Enter with orthophosphate present	Enter with ortho-phosphate and L-malate present	Do not enter
Phosphate	L-Malate	Citrate	Chloride
Arsenate	D-Malate	*cis*-Aconitate	Bromide
Formate	Malonate	Isocitrate	Bicarbonate
Acetate	Isomalate	D-Tartrate	Sulphate
Propionate	Succinate	L-Tartrate	Nitrate
Butyrate	Itaconate	α-Methylmalate	Fumarate[b]
	D-Tartrate	α-Ketoglutarate	Maleate
	meso-Tartrate	α-Ketoadipate	Methylmaleate
	2-Methylsuccinate	Tricarballylate[c]	Methylfumarate
	2,2-Dimethylsuccinate		Dihydroxymaleate
			n-Butylmalonate
			2-Phenylsuccinate
			trans-Aconitate
			Oxaloacetate[b]
			(−)-Hydroxycitrate[c]

[a] Adapted from Chappell[198].
[b] See text, p. 43.
[c] G. R. Williams and B. H. Robinson, private communication.

entity involved in conferring permeability, without implying a mechanistic explanation. That permeases are enzyme-like in nature can be inferred from the high specificity which they exhibit. Table VI lists the specific permeases related to the functioning of the citric acid cycle, which probably exist to facilitate the entry of specific anions into the matrix space of mitochondria. Some of the experimental observations which led to the postulation of these permeases will now be reviewed.

(i) Orthophosphate permease

Of a number of inorganic ions tested, only orthophosphate and arsenate were found to penetrate the inner mitochondrial membrane readily[201]. Chloride and sulfate ions did not penetrate. The ionic diameters of the hydrated ions are: chloride, 2.30 Å; sulfate, 4.40 Å; phosphate monoanion, 4.94 Å; and phosphate dianion, 6.19 Å. The excluded ions are thus smaller than the ions which can pass through the inner mitochondrial membrane. This has been interpreted as implying the existence of a specific phosphate permease which permits passage of phosphate and the closely related arsenate but not of many anions. Chappell and Haarhoff[197] suggest that orthophosphate penetrates as the monoanion by exchanging with a hydroxide ion (Fig. 9).

(ii) Adenine nucleotide permease

Studies by Klingenberg and co-workers[205-209] and by Vignais and co-workers[210,211] have shown that adenine nucleotides enter and leave the mitochondria through the intermediate action of a specific permease which permits passage of adenine nucleotides but not of other nucleotides[207]. The permease exhibits the properties associated with exchange diffusion. Thus, it has been shown by a combination of labeling and rapid separation techniques that the entry into the mitochondria of a molecule of ADP is accompanied by the exit of a molecule of ADP or ATP. The most cogent evidence for the existence in mitochondria of an adenine nucleotide permease comes from the discovery of a specific inhibitor, the compound atractyloside.

Atractyloside is a powerful inhibitor of oxidative phosphorylation in isolated, intact mitochondria. It has no effect on oxidative phosphorylation in submitochondrial particles. It has been shown to block the exchange of intra- and extramitochondrial ADP and ATP.

Recent evidence indicates that in addition to the exchange diffusion of adenine nucleotides, there exists a mechanism which produces an [ATP]/

TABLE VI

THE ANION PERMEASES OF MITOCHONDRIA[a]

Permease specificity	Activators	Inhibitors	Occurrence in mitochondria	Refs.
Phosphate (and arsenate)	None	—	Probably all	201
ATP, ADP		Atractyloside	Probably all	210
Dicarboxylic acids (malate, succinate, but not fumarate)	Phosphate[b]	Butylmalonate	Liver, brain, kidney, heart, *Candida utilis*[c]	197
α-Ketoglutarate	Phosphate[b] + malate, or malonate, but not isomalate	Butylmalonate	Liver, brain, kidney heart, *Candida utilis*[c]	204, 213, 215
Citrate, isocitrate, *cis*-aconitate	Phosphate[b] + malate, or isomalate, but not malonate	Butylmalonate	Liver, kidney, low activity in heart and brain[c]	197, 202, 203, 213
Glutamate	Phosphate (slightly)	4-Hydroxyglutamate; or 2-aminoadipate; or *threo*-hydroxy-aspartate	Liver, kidney, brain, heart	221
Aspartate	Glutamate, or 4-hydroxyglutamate, or 2-aminoadipate; or *threo*-hydroxyaspartate	—	Liver, kidney and heart	221

[a] From Chappell[198].

[b] The requirement for phosphate is apparent mainly in experiments in which swelling in ammonium salts of the anions is measured[197]. In general, phosphate has little effect on the rate of reduction of mitochondrial pyridine nucleotides, unless the substrate-level phosphorylation associated with ketoglutarate oxidation is implicated.

[c] Not present in mitochondria from blow-fly flight muscle.

[ADP] ratio which is considerably greater in the extra- than in the intra-mitochondrial space[209]. This is the opposite of what would be expected from a simple exchange diffusion, since the ratio [ATP]/[ADP] should be greater in the intramitochondrial compartment, where ATP is generated than in the extramitochondrial compartment, where ATP is utilized.

(iii) Dicarboxylic acid permease

In the presence of orthophosphate a number of dicarboxylic acids, including L-malate, D-malate and *meso*-tartrate, penetrate liver mitochondria rapidly. Other dicarboxylic acids, such as fumarate and maleate, do not penetrate the mitochondria[197,198]. It has been suggested that the dicarboxylic acids enter the mitochondrial matrix as dianions by exchanging with orthophosphate[197] (Fig. 9).

The entry of dicarboxylic acids is specifically inhibited by *n*-butylmalonate (pentane-1,1-dicarboxylic acid). For example, *n*-butylmalonate inhibits the oxidation of succinate by intact mitochondria, but not by mitochondria the membranes of which have been ruptured. *n*-Butylmalonate also inhibits the reduction of mitochondrial pyridine nucleotide which occurs when malate is used to facilitate the entry of α-ketoglutarate or isocitrate. The K_i for

Fig. 9. Interrelationship of phosphate, dicarboxylic acid, and tricarboxylic acid permeases of mitochondria. The large circles represent various permeases. The entry of ammonium salts is shown for simplicity. (*i*) *Phosphate permease*. Orthophosphate dianion is shown to become protonated and to enter the matrix space as a monoanion in exchange for a hydroxyl. In the matrix space the monoanion yields the dianion and a proton. Two extra-mitochondrial ammonium ions yield two protons and two ammonias, the two ammonias enter the matrix space and are then protonated. The net effect is the entry of diammonium orthophosphate. (*ii*) *Malate permease*. Malate dianion enters the matrix space in exchange for an orthophosphate dianion. The orthophosphate then reenters the matrix space as described above. Thus orthophosphate acts catalytically in the entry of malate. The net effect is the entry of diammonium malate. (*iii*) *α-Ketoglutarate permease*. A molecule of α-ketoglutarate dianion enters the matrix space in exchange for a malate dianion. The malate then reenters the matrix space as described above. Thus malate and orthophosphate act catalytically in the entry of α-ketoglutarate. The net effect is the entry of diammonium α-ketoglutarate. The evidence for the existence of separate permeases for α-ketoglutarate and other dicarboxylic acids is discussed in the text (see also Table VI). (*iv*) *Tricarboxylic acid permease*. A citrate trianion is shown to become protonated to give the dianion, and to enter the matrix space in exchange for a dicarboxylic acid dianion such as malate. The dicarboxylic acid (for example, malate) then reenters the matrix space as described above. Thus malate and orthophosphate act catalytically in the entry of tricar-boxylic acids. In the matrix space the citrate dianion yields the citrate trianion and a proton. An extramitochondrial ammonium ion yields a proton and ammonia. The latter enters the matrix space and is protonated. The net effect is the entry of triammonium citrate.

n-butylmalonate is about 0.4 mM. It does not inhibit malate, α-ketoglutarate and isocitrate dehydrogenases. A simple hypothesis which fits the observed facts is that n-butylmalonate inhibits the orthophosphate-activated permease (see Table VI), and that inhibition of α-ketoglutarate and isocitrate uptake occurs as a consequence of the inhibition of malate uptake (see below).

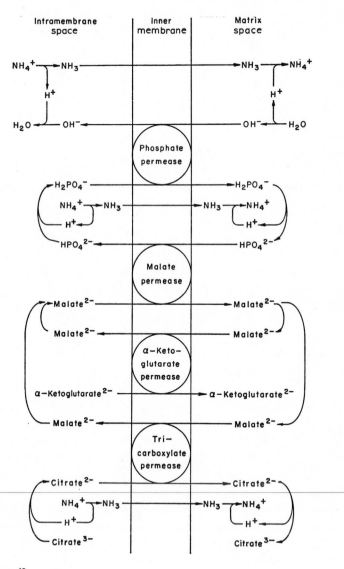

(iv) α-Ketoglutarate permease

In the absence of activators, liver mitochondria are impermeable to α-ketoglutarate Addition of L-malate or certain other dicarboxylic acids such as malonate render the mitochondria permeable. Thus substrate-depleted mitochondria do not metabolize α-ketoglutarate *via* transamination, reductive amination or dehydrogenation unless L-malate or malonate is present[212-217]. It has been proposed that α-ketoglutarate enters the mitochondrial matrix as the dianion by exchange with the malate dianion (Fig. 9).

(v) Tricarboxylic acid permease

Liver mitochondria are impermeable to citrate, isocitrate and *cis*-aconitate unless orthophosphate and malate, or some of the substances listed in Table VI, are present[198,218]. *n*-Butylmalonate acts as a competitive inhibitor with respect to the malate activation of citrate entry[212,213,219]. If mitochondria are first allowed to accumulate malate, and citrate is then added, there is a loss of malate and an uptake of citrate[220]. It has been suggested that tricarboxylic acids enter the mitochondrial matrix as dianions by exchanging with the malate dianion[212,213].

Although the entry of both tricarboxylic acids and α-ketoglutarate is activated by malate, separate permeases appear to be involved. The relative effectiveness of a number of dicarboxylic acids in facilitating the entry of isocitrate and α-ketoglutarate into the matrix of liver mitochondria is shown in Table VII[212]. The results indicate different specificities for the activators of tricarboxylic acid uptake and α-ketoglutarate uptake. Moreover, the α-ketoglutarate permease is very active in heart mitochondria, while the tricarboxylic acid permease is relatively inactive. In liver and kidney mitochondria both permeases are active[198,213].

(vi) Glutamate permease

It has been reported that the pH optimum of glutamate dehydrogenase in intact mitochondria is more acid than the pH optimum of the solubilized enzyme. Moreover, glutamate oxidation by intact mitochondria is competitively inhibited by glutamate analogs, such as α-aminoadipate, which do not inhibit the glutamate dehydrogenase reaction catalyzed by broken liver mitochondria. These observations have been interpreted as indicating the occurrence of a glutamate permease[221]. Other explanations cannot be ruled out at present, and the existence of this permease cannot yet be considered to be firmly established.

(vii) Aspartate permease

When added to intact mitochondria, aspartate does not react in the aspartate aminotransferase reaction unless glutamate or an analog of glutamate is also added. This observation has been interpreted as showing that mitochondria possess a permease for aspartate which requires activation by glutamate[221]. It is assumed that glutamate can enter the matrix space as a monoanion by exchange with a hydroxide anion, and that glutamate or one of its analogs then exchanges with aspartate.

(viii) Entry of fumarate and oxaloacetate

There appears to be no permease which permits the transfer across the inner mitochondrial membrane of fumarate. Furthermore, there is doubt whether oxaloacetate is able to penetrate the inner mitochondrial membrane. The question of oxaloacetate uptake and egress is somewhat controversial. The intracellular levels of oxaloacetate are very low. Calculations based on the ratios of concentrations [NADH]/[NAD] in the cytoplasm and the mitochondrial matrix, and on the total malate and oxaloacetate of liver show the intracellular distribution of oxaloacetate to be very skew. The concentration of oxaloacetate in the cytoplasm and in the mitochondrial matrix has been calculated to be about 10 μM and 0.1–0.5 μM, respectively, in the case of rat liver[222]. The concentration gradient of oxaloacetate would appear to favor a flow of this substance into the mitochondria. However, the uptake of low (10 μM) concentrations of oxaloacetate into the mitochondrial matrix is very slow unless a source of energy and a cation such as K^+, which enters the matrix by an energy-linked process, is provided[223-225]. The inference is that oxaloacetate enters passively as a counter ion to the energy-linked uptake of cations. This possibility is discussed below in more detail in connection with the energy-linked uptake by mitochondria of other members of the citric acid cycle.

(ix) Mitochondria from flight muscle of insects

Most of the permeases listed in Table VI are absent from mitochondria prepared from flight muscle of insects. Mitochondria from this source oxidize only two externally added substrates rapidly, namely pyruvate and α-glycerophosphate. They are also capable of oxidizing proline at about 10% the rate of α-glycerophosphate oxidation[199]. It has been suggested that this is probably a consequence of the single-purpose role of these mitochondria: the aerobic synthesis of ATP from ADP[198,226]. Liver mitochondria possess a much more complex metabolic role; for example, they participate in the synthesis of phosphoenolpyruvate, in the reductive amination of α-ketoglutarate, in urea synthesis, and in the synthesis of various amino acids, in addition to possessing the enzymes of the citric acid cycle and of oxidative phosphorylation. As a corollary, liver mitochondria seem to possess a complex complement of anion permeases.

(x) Energy-linked uptake of anions

Liver mitochondria possess the capacity to take up citrate[227,228]. The citrate is accumulated in the matrix space since it is not removed by washing with isotonic sucrose. Citrate uptake is prevented by inhibitors of respiration,

TABLE VII

STIMULATION OF ISOCITRATE AND α-KETOGLUTARATE ENTRY BY
DICARBOXYLIC ACIDS

Rat liver mitochondria were suspended in 0.1 M KCl containing 20 mM Tris–HCl, and 1 mM phosphate, both at pH 7.2. The mitochondria were incubated with 1 mM fluorocarbonylcyanidephenylhydrazone at 30° for 30 min to deplete them of endogenous substrates. Then antimycin (0.16 μg/ml) followed by 1 mM isocitrate or 1 mM oxoglutarate was added. The rate of reduction of intramitochondrial pyridine nucleotides on addition of 1 mM of the compounds listed was followed at 340–373 mμ by double-beam spectrophotometry. All rates are referred to L-malate as 100. (From Chappell and Robinson[212].)

Compound	Isocitrate entry	α-Ketoglutarate entry
L-Malate	100	100
Maleate	28	74
Malonate	0	56
meso-Tartrate	17	46
Succinate	17	46
Itaconate (2-methylenesuccinate)	28	25
Citraconate (2-methylmaleate)	0	9
D,L-2-Methylsuccinate	0	9
D-Malate	6	7
D-Tartrate	0	0
L-Tartrate	0	0
Tartronate (2-hydroxymalonate)	50	5
Isomalate (2-hydroxy-2-methylmalonate)	53	8
2,2-Dimethylmalonate	20	17

such as rotenone and antimycin, and by uncouplers of oxidative phosphorylation, such as dinitrophenol. The process thus appears to be "energy-linked"[229,230]. The uptake of citrate is not prevented by oligomycin, which blocks ATP synthesis without affecting the formation of the energy-rich intermediates of oxidative phosphorylation. It is supported by ATP when respiration is inhibited by antimycin. Under these conditions citrate uptake is inhibited by oligomycin, presumably because this substance prevents the generation from ATP of the energy-rich intermediates which are involved in the accumulation process.

The energy-linked uptake of citrate shows a requirement for a dicarboxylic acid such as malate[230]. This indicates that tricarboxylate permease is involved in the uptake of citrate even when the process is energy-dependent.

The general properties described for citrate uptake coincide with those observed for *cation* uptake. It might be concluded that citrate is accumulated passively through the tricarboxylic acid permease as a counter-ion to the "active" uptake of a cation such as potassium. This possibility was discounted since no dependence on any particular cation could be observed[229]. Citrate accumulation occurs in the absence of added potassium and magnesium ions and in the presence of 1 mM EDTA; and it has been shown that citrate accumulation is not linked to changes in the content of mitochondrial potassium and magnesium ions[229,231]. However, as has been stressed by Greville[200], metal ion participation is difficult to disprove. Anion uptake may depend on the repeated movement into and out of the mitochondria of the small amount of endogenous potassium ion in the mitochondrial preparation. Greville has pointed out another possibility: that an anion enters the mitochondrial matrix together with a proton, the anion–proton symport of Mitchell[232]. Put differently, an anion enters in exchange for the exit of a hydroxide ion. The latter process cannot be distinguished from anion entry with a proton. In either case the accumulation is linked to a respiration-dependent proton ejection. Proton ejection from the matrix provides an excess of hydroxide ion in the matrix, which can promote anion accumulation by exchange of anion with hydroxide ion[200].

Studies of the uptake of malate, succinate and glutamate by liver mitochondria have thrown further light on the role played by the cation. In the presence of potassium ions the uptake of these dicarboxylic acids was greatly enhanced by adding valinomycin or gramicidin[233,234] or nonactin[235]. These substances have been shown to stimulate the energy-linked uptake of potassium ions by mitochondria[236,237]. Nigericin causes the loss of potassium ions accumulated by mitochondria in the presence of valinomycin[238, 239]; it causes the discharge of anions accumulated with potassium ions[240, 241]. In this case too, the uptake of the anions was prevented by inhibitors of respiration and by uncouplers of oxidative phosphorylation. Since respiratory inhibitors and uncouplers prevent uptake of cations, it was concluded that the anions are taken up passively with cations[233]. However, anion and cation may have a linked energy dependence so that the uptake of neither can strictly be regarded as passive[234,242].

The cytoplasmic potassium ion concentration, about 80–120 mM, is in the same range as that estimated to exist in the mitochondrial matrix. This would seem to render superfluous an energy-dependent potassium ion pumping mechanism in the inner membrane. This point has led Pressman and associates to propose that the function of the cation pump in mitochondria is to drive and control the anion flux into and out of the mitochondrial matrix[243,244]. Studies which cannot be gone into here lend support to this proposal[245,246].

TABLE VIII

RELATION BETWEEN POTASSIUM ION AND SUBSTRATE ANION CONTENT IN RAT LIVER MITOCHONDRIA

Mitochondria (9.2 mg protein per ml) were incubated in 50 mM sucrose, 25 mM Tris–HCl buffer, 25 mM KCl, 5 mM MgCl$_2$, 2 mM EDTA, 1 mM sodium arsenite. 1 μg per ml rotenone, 4 μg per ml antimycin, and substrate in the concentration range of 0.5 to 5.0 mM. The final pH was 7.4, and the temperature was room temperature. The medium also contained 0.2 μCi per ml ^{3}H$_2$O and 0.5 μCi per ml [^{14}C] substrate. Samples of 0.2 ml were withdrawn at appropriate intervals, centrifuged through silicone, and assayed for radioactivity and potassium. Substrate and potassium accumulation in the matrix was then calculated, including appropriate corrections for the sucrose-permeable space which were determined in a parallel experiment[247].

Substrate	Apparent K_m for substrate uptake (mM)	Maximum amount of substrate in matrix (mM)	Amount of K$^+$ in matrix when substrate content is maximum (mequiv.)
Succinate	1.5	45	121
Malate	1.7	36	84
Malonate	1.3	30	90
α-Ketoglutarate	2.5	50	156
Citrate	1.3	36	90
Pyruvate	6.3	100	106
Glutamate	4.5	50	126
β-Hydroxybutyrate	4.5	35	59

Considerable caution must be exercised in deciding whether the accumulation of an anion is or is not energy-linked. For example, both malate and succinate may supply energy in the form of the energy-rich intermediates of oxidative phosphorylation and ion transport, even in the presence of various inhibitors. However, rotenone blocks the generation of energy-rich intermediates from malate, while antimycin fulfills the same function for succinate. In the presence of these inhibitors malate and succinate will still act as permease activators, but energy must now be provided in some other form to bring about anion accumulation[231].

Although the maximum amount of potassium ions accumulated by mitochondria *in vitro* varies somewhat from preparation to preparation, the maximum concentration of substrate accumulated approaches the equivalent potassium ion concentration in the matrix (Table VIII). This suggests that although the concentration of substrate anion may rise greatly over the extramitochondrial concentration of the anion, its level is ultimately limited by the positive charges available in the mitochondrion. The excess of potassium ion probably serves to neutralize various fixed negative charges within the mitochondrion[247]. The concept that the cation level limits the anion level in mitochondria is supported by competition experiments in which two different anions were allowed to accumulate in the presence of each other. Competition was observed in the sense that the amount of one anion accumulated by mitochondria limited the amount of another type of anion which was accumulated[230,247].

(xi) General comments

It has been pointed out by Greville[200] that even if anions are taken *up* against a concentration gradient, expenditure of energy may not be necessary, provided that the emergent anions are passing *down* a concentration gradient. The thermodynamic purist may feel that this statement is true only if the system is perfectly reversible.

During the uptake of ions, electrical neutrality must be maintained. As has been stressed by Slater[248], this means that the uptake of anions is accompanied by either (a) uptake of an equivalent amount of cation, or (b) the extrusion of an equivalent amount of endogenous anion. In the case of (a) the osmotic pressure in the matrix will increase, and the mitochondria will swell; in (b) the osmotic pressure will remain unchanged, and no swelling will occur.

Slater[248] has discussed a somewhat more complex scheme for the uptake of ammonium succinate than that shown in Fig. 9. It differs from Fig. 9 in that each kind of substrate anion entering or leaving the mitochondrial matrix does so in exchange for one or two hydroxide ions. Even the energy-linked uptake of a cation such as Ca^{2+} is postulated to involve the simultaneous output of H^+ and OH^-; the OH^- output being accompanied by an uptake of an anion such as succinate.

The permeases described in this section presumably exist for the purpose of controlling the flow of metabolites across the mitochondrial membrane. The permeability of the membrane to citric acid cycle and related anions shows a complex interdependence which is clearly of significance to the regulation of the citric acid cycle in general and to the intra- and extramitochondrial portions of the cycle in particular. However, our understanding of the anion permeases is still very limited, and it is not yet possible to fit their detailed functions into a complete description of the operation and control of the citric acid cycle in the intact cell.

REFERENCES

1 S. KORKES, J. R. STERN, I. C. GUNSALUS AND S. OCHOA, *Nature*, 166 (1950) 439; S. KORKES, A. DEL CAMPILLO, I. C. GUNSALUS AND S. OCHOA, *J. Biol. Chem.*, 193 (1951) 721; S. KORKES, in W. D. MCELROY AND B. GLASS (Eds.), *Phosphorus Metabolism*, Vol. 1, Johns Hopkins, Baltimore, Md., 1951, p. 259.
2 R. S. SCHWEET, M. FULD, K. CHESLOCK AND M. H. PAUL, in W. D. MCELROY AND B. GLASS (Eds.), *Phosphorus Metabolism*, Vol. 1, Johns Hopkins, Baltimore, Md., 1951, p. 246.
3 D. R. SANADI, J. W. LITTLEFIELD AND R. M. BOCK, *J. Biol. Chem.*, 197 (1952) 851.
4 I. C. GUNSALUS, in W. D. MCELROY AND B. GLASS (Eds.), *Symposium on the Mechanism of Enzyme Action*, Johns Hopkins, Baltimore, Md., 1954, p. 545; *Federation Proc.*, 13 (1954) 715.
5 L. J. REED, *Advan. Enzymol.*, 18 (1957) 319.
6 D. R. SANADI, in P. D. BOYER, H. LARDY AND K. MYRBÄCK (Eds.), *The Enzymes*, Vol. 7, Academic Press, New York, 1963, p. 307.
7 V. MASSEY, in P. D. BOYER, H. LARDY AND K. MYRBÄCK (Eds.), *The Enzymes*, Vol. 7, Academic Press, New York, 1963, p. 275.
8 L. J. REED, in M. FLORKIN AND E. H. STOTZ (Eds.), *Comprehensive Biochemistry*, Vol. 14, Elsevier, Amsterdam, 1966, p. 99.
9 H. J. STRECKER AND S. OCHOA, *J. Biol. Chem.*, 209 (1954) 313.
10 S. KORKES, *Brookhaven Symp. Biol.*, 5 (1952) 192.
11 M. GOLDBERG AND D. R. SANADI, *J. Am. Chem. Soc.*, 74 (1952) 4972.
12 A. D. GOUNARIS AND L. P. HAGER, *J. Biol. Chem.*, 236 (1961) 1013.
13 M. KOIKE, L. J. REED AND W. R. CARROLL, *J. Biol. Chem.*, 238 (1963) 30.
14 M. KOIKE AND L. J. REED, *J. Biol. Chem.*, 235 (1960) 1931.
15 M. L. DAS, M. KOIKE AND L. J. REED, *Proc. Natl. Acad. Sci. (U.S.)*, 47 (1961) 753.
16 V. MASSEY, *Biochim. Biophys. Acta*, 38 (1960) 447.
17 R. BRESLOW, *J. Am. Chem. Soc.*, 80 (1958) 3719.
18 R. BRESLOW, *Ann. N. Y. Acad. Sci.*, 98 (1962) 445.
19 L. O. KRAMPITZ, I. SUZUKI AND G. GREULL, *Ann. N.Y. Acad. Sci.*, 98 (1962) 466.
20 L. O. KRAMPITZ, I. SUZUKI AND G. GREULL, *Brookhaven Symp. Biol.*, 15 (1962) 282.
21 P. SCRIBA AND H. HOLZER, *Biochem. Z.*, 334 (1961) 473.
22 H. HOLZER, F. DA FONSECA-WOLLHEIM, G. KOHLHAW AND C. W. WOENCKHAUS, *Ann. N.Y. Acad. Sci.*, 98 (1962) 453.
23 H. W. GOEDDE, K. G. BLUME AND H. HOLZER, *Biochim. Biophys. Acta*, 62 (1962) 1.
24 H. W. GOEDDE, B. ULRICH, C. STAHLMANN AND H. HOLZER, *Biochem. Z.*, 343 (1965) 204.
25 J. ULLRICH AND A. MANNSCHRECK, *Biochim. Biophys. Acta*, 115 (1966) 46.
26 A. SCHELLENBERG, A. KOLBE AND G. HÜBNER, *Z. Physiol. Chem.*, 341 (1965) 22.
27 D. R. SANADI, M. LANGLEY AND F. WHITE, *J. Biol. Chem.*, 234 (1959) 183.
28 O. K. REISS, *J. Biol. Chem.*, 233 (1958) 789.
29 D. R. SANADI, M. LANGLEY AND F. WHITE, *Biochim. Biophys. Acta*, 29 (1958) 218.
30 L. J. REED, R. F. LEACH AND M. KOIKE, *J. Biol. Chem.*, 232 (1958) 123.
31 L. J. REED, M. KOIKE, M. E. LEVITCH AND R. F. LEACH, *J. Biol. Chem.*, 232 (1958) 143.
32 H. NAWA, W. T. BRADY, M. KOIKE AND L. J. REED, *J. Am. Chem. Soc.*, 82 (1960) 896.
33 I. C. GUNSALUS, L. S. BARTON AND W. GRUBER, *J. Am. Chem. Soc.*, 78 (1956) 1763.
34 V. MASSEY, in W. A. WOOD (Ed.), *Methods in Enzymology*, Vol. 9, Academic Press, New York, 1966, p. 272.

35   D. R. Sanadi, M. Langley and R. L. Searls, *J. Biol. Chem.*, 234 (1959) 178.
36   R. L. Searls and D. R. Sanadi, *J. Biol. Chem.*, 235 (1960) 2485.
37   V. Massey, Q. H. Gibson and C. Veeger, *Biochem. J.*, 77 (1960) 341.
38   V. Massey and C. Veeger, *Biochim. Biophys. Acta*, 48 (1961) 33.
39   R. L. Searls, J. M. Peeters and D. R. Sanadi, *J. Biol. Chem.*, 236 (1961) 2317.
40   G. Palmer and V. Massey, *Biochim. Biophys. Acta*, 58 (1962) 349.
41   F. B. Straub, *Biochem. J.*, 33 (1939) 787.
41   V. Massey, *Biochim. Biophys. Acta*, 30 (1958) 205.
43   R. L. Searls and D. R. Sanadi, *J. Biol. Chem.*, 236 (1961) 580.
44   L. J. Reed and D. J. Cox, *Ann. Rev. Biochem.*, 35 (1966) 57.
45   L. J. Reed and R. M. Oliver, *Brookhaven Symp. Biol.*, 21 (1968) 397.
46   M. Koike, L. J. Reed and W. R. Carroll, *J. Biol. Chem.*, 235 (1960) 1924.
47   C. R. Willms, R. M. Oliver, H. R. Henney, B. B. Mukherjee and L. J. Reed, *J. Biol. Chem.*, 242 (1967) 889.
48   V. Jagannathan and R. S. Schweet, *J. Biol. Chem.*, 196 (1962) 551.
49   R. S. Schweet, B. Katchman, R. M. Bock and V. Jagannathan, *J. Biol. Chem.*, 196 (1952) 563.
50   T. Hayakawa, M. Hirashima, S. Ide, M. Hamada, K. Okabe and M. Koike, *J. Biol. Chem.*, 241 (1966) 4694.
51   E. Ishikawa, R. M. Oliver and L. J. Reed, *Proc. Natl. Acad. Sci. (U.S.)*, 56 (1966) 534.
52   M. Hirashima, T. Hayakawa and M. Koike, *J. Biol. Chem.*, 242 (1967) 902.
53   T. Hayakawa and M. Koike, *J. Biol. Chem.*, 242 (1967) 1356.
54   C. J. Lusty and T. P. Singer, *J. Biol. Chem.*, 239 (1964) 3733.
55   D. R. Sanadi, personal communication.
56   U. Henning, C. Herz and K. Szolyvay, *Z. Vererbungslehre*, 95 (1964) 236.
57   T. C. Linn, F. H. Pettit and L. J. Reed, *Proc. Natl. Acad. Sci. (U.S.)*, 62 (1969) 234.
58   E. G. Krebs, R. J. DeLange, R. G. Kemp and W. D. Riley, *Pharmacol. Rev.*, 18 (1966) 163.
59   F. Huijing and J. Larner, *Proc. Natl. Acad. Sci. (U.S.)*, 56 (1966) 647.
60   P. B. Garland, E. A. Newsholme and P. J. Randle, *Nature*, 195 (1962) 381.
61   J. Bremer, *Biochim. Biophys. Acta*, 104 (1963) 581.
62   G. V. Jagow, B. Westermann and O. Wieland, *Eur. J. Biochem.*, 3 (1968) 512.
63   P. B. Garland and P. J. Randle, *Biochem. J.*, 91 (1964) 6c.
64   R. G. Hansen and H. V. Henning, *Biochim. Biophys. Acta*, 122 (1966) 355.
65   E. R. Schwarz and L. J. Reed, *Federation Proc.*, 27 (1968) 389.
66   E. R. Schwarz, L. O. Old and L. J. Reed, *Biochem. Biophys. Res. Commun.*, 31 (1968) 495.
67   P. B. Garland, D. Shepherd, D. G. Nicholls, D. W. Yates and P. A. Light, in J. M. Lowenstein (Ed.), *Citric Acid Cycle. Control and Compartmentation*, Marcel Dekker, New York, 1969, p. 163.
68   H. A. Krebs, *Proc. Roy. Soc. (London)*, B, 159 (1964) 545.
69   M. C. Scrutton and M. F. Utter, *Ann. Rev. Biochem.*, 37 (1968) 249.
70   J. Bremer, *Biochim. Biophys. Acta*, 116 (1966) 1.
71   D. G. Nicholls, D. Shepherd and P. B. Garland, *Biochem. J.*, 103 (1967) 677.
72   H. D. Söling, B. Willms, D. Friedrichs and J. Kleinecke, *Eur. J. Biochem.*, 4 (1968) 364.
73   E. Struck, J. Ashmore and O. Wieland, *Biochem. Z.*, 343 (1965) 107.
74   J. R. Williamson, R. A. Kreisberg and P. W. Felts, *Proc. Natl. Acad. Sci. (U.S.)*, 56 (1966) 247.

75 H. TEUFEL, L. A. MENAHAN, J. C. SHIPP, S. BÖNING AND O. WIELAND, *Eur. J. Biochem.*, 2 (1967) 182.
76 M. G. HERRERA, D. KAMM, N. RUDERMANN AND G. F. CAHILL JR., *Advan. Enzyme Regulation*, 4 (1966) 225.
77 M. F. UTTER AND D. B. KEECH, *J. Biol. Chem.*, 235 (1960) PC 17.
78 P. B. GARLAND, D. SHEPHERD AND D. W. YATES, *Biochem. J.*, 97 (1965) 587.
79 H. A. KREBS AND W. A. JOHNSON, *Enzymologia*, 4 (1937) 148. (Note: This paper has recently been reprinted in J. M. LOWENSTEIN (Ed.), *Citric Acid Cycle. Control and Compartmentation*, Marcel Dekker, New York, 1969, p. xiii.)
80 H. A. KREBS, in D. M. GREENBERG (Ed.), *Chemical Pathways of Metabolism (1st ed.)*, Vol. 1, Academic Press, New York, 1954, p. 109.
81 H. A. KREBS AND J. M. LOWENSTEIN, in D. M. GREENBERG (Ed.), *Metabolic Pathways (2nd ed.)*, Vol. 1, Academic Press, New York, 1960, p. 129.
82 J. M. LOWENSTEIN, in D. M. GREENBERG (Ed.), *Metabolic Pathways (3rd ed.)*, Vol. 1, Academic Press, New York, 1967, p. 146.
83 H. KREBS, in H. N. MUNRO AND J. B. ALLISON (Eds.), *Mammalian Protein Metabolism*, Vol. 1, Academic Press, New York, 1964, p. 125.
84 J. M. LOWENSTEIN (Ed.), *Methods in Enzymology*, Vol. 13, Academic Press, New York, 1969.
85 A. L. LEHNINGER, *The Mitochondrion*, Benjamin, New York, 1964.
86 G. D. GREVILLE, in J. M. LOWENSTEIN (Ed.), *Citric Acid Cycle. Control and Compartmentation*, Marcel Dekker, New York, 1969, p. 1.
87 V. P. WHITTAKER, in J. M. TAGER, S. PAPA, E. QUAGLIARIELLO AND E. C. SLATER (Eds.), *Regulation of Metabolic Processes in Mitochondria (BBA Library, Vol. 7)*, Elsevier, Amsterdam, 1966, p. 1.
88 C. ROUILLER, *Intern. Rev. Cytol.*, 9 (1960) 227.
89 A. B. NOVIKOFF, in J. BRACHET AND A. E. MIRSKY (Eds.), *The Cell*, Vol. 2, Academic Press, New York, 1961, p. 299.
90 D. F. PARSON, *Intern. Rev. Exptl. Pathol.*, 4 (1965) 1.
91 D. E. GREEN, W. F. LOOMIS AND V. H. AUERBACH, *J. Biol. Chem.*, 172 (1948) 389.
92 W. C. SCHNEIDER AND V. R. POTTER, *J. Biol. Chem.*, 177 (1949) 893.
93 E. P. KENNEDY AND A. L. LEHNINGER, *J. Biol. Chem.*, 179 (1949) 957.
94 D. E. GREEN, *J. Cellular Comp. Physiol.*, 39, *Suppl.* 2 (1952) 75.
95 W. C. SCHNEIDER AND G. H. HOGEBOOM, *Cancer Res.*, 11 (1951) 1.
96 W. C. SCHNEIDER, *Advan. Enzymol.*, 21 (1959) 1.
97 C. DE DUVE, R. WATTIAUX AND P. BAUDHUIN, *Advan. Enzymol.*, 24 (1962) 291.
98 C. DE DUVE, *J. Theoret. Biol.*, 6 (1964) 33.
99 C. DE DUVE, *Harvey Lectures Ser.*, 59 (1965) 49.
100 D. B. ROODYN, *Intern. Rev. Cytol.*, 18 (1965) 99.
101 E. ZEBE, *Biochem. Z.*, 332 (1960) 328.
102 P. A. SRERE AND G. W. KOSICKI, *J. Biol. Chem.*, 236 (1961) 2557.
103 D. PETTE, in J. M. TAGER, S. PAPA, E. QUAGLIARIELLO AND E. C. SLATER (Eds.), *Regulation of Metabolic Processes in Mitochondria (BBA Library, Vol. 7)*, Elsevier, Amsterdam, 1966, p. 28.
104 P. A. SRERE, *J. Biol. Chem.*, 234 (1959) 2544.
105 S. R. DICKMAN AND J. F. SPEYER, *J. Biol. Chem.*, 206 (1954) 67.
106 J. A. SHEPHERD AND G. KALNITSKY, *J. Biol. Chem.*, 207 (1954) 605.
107 J. A. SHEPHERD, Y. W. LI, E. E. MASON AND S. E. ZIFFREN, *J. Biol. Chem.*, 213 (1955) 405.
108 M. R. V. MURTHY AND D. A. RAPPOPORT, *Biochim. Biophys. Acta*, 74 (1963) 51.
109 W. R. FRISELL, M. V. PATWARDHAN AND C. G. MACKENZIE, *J. Biol. Chem.*, 240 (1965) 1829.

110   J. L. PURVIS, *Biochim. Biophys. Acta*, 30 (1958) 440.
111   G. W. E. PLAUT AND S. C. SUNG, *J. Biol. Chem.*, 207 (1954) 305.
112   L. ERNSTER AND F. NAVAZIO, *Exptl. Cell Res.*, 11 (1956) 483.
113   J. L. BELL AND D. N. BARON, *Biochem. J.*, 90 (1964) 8P.
114   H. GOEBELL AND D. PETTE, *Enzymol. Biol. Clin.*, 8 (1967) 161.
115   A. DELBRÜCK, H. SCHIMASSEK, K. BARTSCH AND T. BÜCHER, *Biochem. Z.*, 331 (1959) 297.
116   J. A. SHEPHERD, *J. Histochem. Cytochem.*, 4 (1956) 47.
117   J. A. SHEPHERD, *J. Histochem. Cytochem.*, 9 (1961) 528.
118   G. H. HOGEBOOM AND W. C. SCHNEIDER, *J. Biol. Chem.*, 186 (1950) 417.
119   G. W. E. PLAUT AND K. A. PLAUT, *J. Biol. Chem.*, 199 (1952) 141.
120   L. ERNSTER, *Biochem. Soc. Symp. (Cambridge, Engl.)*, 16 (1959) 54.
121   L. ERNSTER AND F. NAVAZIO, *Acta Chem. Scand.*, 10 (1956) 1038.
122   J. M. LOWENSTEIN AND S. R. SMITH, *Biochim. Biophys. Acta*, 56 (1962) 385.
123   C. DE DUVE AND P. BAUDHUIN, *Physiol. Rev.*, 46 (1966) 323.
124   M. MÜLLER, P. BAUDHUIN AND C. DE DUVE, *J. Cell. Physiol.*, 68 (1966) 165.
125   M. MÜLLER, J. F. HOGG AND C. DE DUVE, *J. Biol. Chem.*, 243 (1968) 5385.
126   J. F. HOGG AND H. L. KORNBERG, *Biochem. J.*, 86 (1963) 462.
127   F. LEIGHTON, B. POOLE, H. BEAUFAY, P. BAUDHUIN, J. W. COFFEY, S. FOWLER AND C. DE DUVE, *J. Cell Biol.*, 37 (1968) 482.
128   R. W. BREIDENBACH AND H. BEEVERS, *Biochem. Biophys. Res. Commun.*, 27 (1967) 462.
129   P. SIEKEVITZ, *J. Biol. Chem.*, 195 (1952) 549.
130   K. W. CLELAND AND E. C. SLATER, *Biochem. J.*, 53 (1953) 547.
131   B. MANDULA, *Thesis*, Brandeis University, 1969.
132   T. E. KING, *Advan. Enzymol.*, 28 (1966) 155.
133   T. P. SINGER AND E. B. KEARNEY, in P. D. BOYER, H. LARDY AND K. MYRBÄCK (Eds.) *The Enzymes (2nd ed.)*, Vol. 7, Academic Press, New York, 1963, p. 383.
134   T. P. SINGER, E. B. KEARNEY AND V. MASSEY, *Advan. Enzymol.*, 18 (1957) 65.
135   O. ARRIGONI AND T. P. SINGER, *Nature*, 193 (1962) 1256.
136   T. F. SLATER AND D. N. PLANTEROSE, *Biochem. J.*, 74 (1960) 584.
137   H. R. MAHLER, M. H. WITTENBERGER AND L. BRAND, *J. Biol. Chem.*, 233 (1958) 770.
138   T. E. KING, in R. W. ESTABROOK AND M. E. PULLMAN (Eds.), *Methods in Enzymology* Vol. 10, Academic Press, New York, 1967, p. 322.
139   C. VEEGER, D. V. DERVARTANIAN AND W. P. ZEYLEMAKER, in J. M. LOWENSTEIN (Ed.), *Methods in Enzymology*, Vol. 13, Academic Press, New York, 1969, p. 81.
140   E. L. KUFF, *J. Biol. Chem.*, 207 (1954) 361.
141   C. DE DUVE, B. C. PRESSMAN, R. GIANETTO, R. WATTIAUX AND F. APPELMANS, *Biochem. J.*, 60 (1955) 604.
142   G. S. CHRISTIE AND S. D. JUDAH, *Proc. Roy. Soc. (London)*, Ser. B, 141 (1954) 420.
143   H. BEAUFAY, D. S. BENDALL, P. BAUDHUIN AND C. DE DUVE, *Biochem. J.*, 73 (1959) 623.
144   L. SIEGEL AND S. ENGLARD, *Biochim. Biophys. Acta*, 54 (1961) 67.
145   B. K. JOYCE AND S. GRISOLIA, *J. Biol. Chem.*, 236 (1961) 725.
146   L. SIEGEL AND S. ENGLARD, *Biochim. Biophys. Acta*, 64 (1962) 101.
147   D. B. ROODYN, J. W. SUTTIE AND T. S. WORK, *Biochem. J.*, 83 (1962) 29.
148   S. ENGLARD AND L. SIEGEL, in J. M. LOWENSTEIN (Ed.), *Methods in Enzymology*, Vol. 13, Academic Press, New York, 1969, p. 99.
149   G. B. KITTO, in J. M. LOWENSTEIN (Ed.), *Methods in Enzymology*, Vol. 13, Academic Press, New York, 1969, p. 106.

150 D. DUPOURQUE AND E. KUN, in J. M. LOWENSTEIN (Ed.), *Methods in Enzymology*, Vol. 13, Academic Press, New York, 1969, p. 116.
151 S. ENGLARD, in J. M. LOWENSTEIN (Ed.), *Methods in Enzymology*, Vol. 13, Academic Press, New York, 1969, p. 123.
152 R. K. GERDING AND R. G. WOLFE, *J. Biol. Chem.*, 244 (1969) 1164.
153 K. D. MUNKRES AND F. M. RICHARDS, *Arch. Biochem. Biophys.*, 109 (1965) 466.
154 A. YOSHIDA, *J. Biol. Chem.*, 240 (1965) 1113.
155 F. C. GRIMM AND D. G. DOHERTY, *J. Biol. Chem.*, 236 (1961) 1980.
156 S. ENGLARD AND H. H. BREIGER, *Biochim. Biophys. Acta*, 56 (1962) 571.
157 C. J. R. THORNE, *Biochim. Biophys. Acta*, 59 (1962) 624.
158 C. J. R. THORNE AND P. M. COOPER, *Biochim. Biophys. Acta*, 81 (1964) 397.
159 G. B. KITTO AND N. O. KAPLAN, *Biochemistry*, 5 (1966) 3966.
160 C. J. R. THORNE AND N. O. KAPLAN, *J. Biol. Chem.*, 238 (1963) 1861.
161 G. B. KITTO AND R. G. LEWIS, *Biochim. Biophys. Acta*, 139 (1967) 1.
162 T.-L. CHAN AND K. A. SCHELLENBERG, *J. Biol. Chem.*, 243 (1968) 6284.
163 D. D. DAVIES, in J. M. LOWENSTEIN (Ed.), *Methods in Enzymology*, Vol. 13, Academic Press, New York, 1969, p. 148.
164 G. B. KITTO, M. E. KOTTKE, L. H. BERTLAND, W. H. MURPHEY and N. O. KAPLAN, *Arch. Biochem. Biophys.*, 121 (1967) 224.
165 A. YOSHIDA, in J. M. LOWENSTEIN (Ed.), *Methods in Enzymology*, Vol. 13, Academic Press, New York, 1969, p. 141.
166 W. H. MURPHEY, C. BARNABY, F. J. LIN and N. O. KAPLAN, *J. Biol. Chem.*, 242 (1967) 1548.
167 W. H. MURPHEY AND G. B. KITTO, in J. M. LOWENSTEIN (Ed.), *Methods in Enzymology*, Vol. 13, Academic Press, New York, 1969, p. 145.
168 L. D. KOHN AND W. B. JACOBY, *J. Biol. Chem.*, 243 (1968) 2472.
169 M. BENZIMAN, in J. M. LOWENSTEIN (Ed.), *Methods in Enzymology*, Vol. 13, Academic Press, New York, 1969, p. 129.
170 P. J. R. PHIZACKERLEY, in J. M. LOWENSTEIN (Ed.), *Methods in Enzymology*, Vol. 13, Academic Press, New York, 1969, p. 135.
171 A. DELBRÜCK, H. SCHIMASSEK, K. BARTSCH AND TH. BÜCHER, *Biochem. Z.*, 331 (1959) 297.
172 J. W. BOYD, *Biochem. J.*, 81 (1961) 434.
173 J. W. BOYD, *Biochem. J.*, 84 (1962) 14P.
174 P. P. COHEN AND H. J. SALLACH, in D. M. GREENBERG (Ed.), *Metabolic Pathways*, Vol. 2, Academic Press, New York, 1961, p. 1.
175 Y. MORINO, H. ITOH AND H. WADA, *Biochem. Biophys. Res. Commun.*, 13 (1963) 348.
176 M. M. BHARGAVA AND A. SREENIVASAN, *Biochem. J.*, 108 (1968) 619.
177 D. PETTE AND W. LUH, *Biochem. Biophys. Res. Commun.*, 8 (1962) 283.
178 W. J. RUTTER AND H. A. LARDY, *J. Biol. Chem.*, 233 (1958) 374.
179 L. SALGANICOFF AND R. E. KOEPPE, *J. Biol. Chem.*, 243 (1968) 3416.
180 H. A. LARDY, D. O. FOSTER, J. W. YOUNG, E. SHRAGO AND P. D. DAZ, *J. Cell. Comp. Physiol.*, 66, *Suppl.* 1 (1965) 39.
181 N. S. HENDERSON, *Arch. Biochem. Biophys.*, 117 (1966) 28.
182 D. B. KEECH AND M. F. UTTER, *J. Biol. Chem.*, 238 (1963) 2609.
183 H. V. HENNING AND W. SEUBERT, *Biochem. Z.*, 340 (1964) 160.
184 H. V. HENNING, B. STUMPF, B. OHLY AND W. SEUBERT, *Biochem. Z.*, 344 (1966) 274.
185 L. RESHEF, F. J. BALLARD AND R. W. HANSON, *J. Biol. Chem.*, 244 (1969) 1994.
186 I. BÖTTGER, O. WIELAND, D. BRDICZKA AND D. PETTE, *Eur. J. Biochem.*, 8 (1969) 113.
187 F. J. BALLARD AND R. W. HANSON, *Biochem. J.*, 104 (1967) 866.
188 F. J. BALLARD AND R. W. HANSON, *J. Lipid Res.*, 8 (1967) 73.

189   B. GUL AND R. DILS, *Biochem. J.*, 111 (1969) 263.
190   R. C. NORDLIE AND H. A. LARDY, *J. Biol. Chem.*, 238 (1963) 2259.
191   W. GEVERS, *Biochem. J.*, 103 (1967) 141.
192   D. D. HOLTEN AND R. C. NORDLIE, *Biochemistry*, 4 (1965) 723.
193   F. J. BALLARD AND R. W. HANSON, *J. Biol. Chem.*, 244 (1969) 5625.
194   F. J. BALLARD, R. W. HANSON AND G. A. LEVEILLE, *J. Biol. Chem.*, 242 (1967) 2746.
195   A. L. LEHNINGER, *Harvey Lectures Ser.*, 49 (1955) 176.
196   J. L. PURVIS AND J. M. LOWENSTEIN, *J. Biol. Chem.*, 236 (1961) 2794.
197   J. B. CHAPPELL AND K. N. HAARHOFF, in E. C. SLATER, Z. KANIUGA AND L. WOJTCZAK (Eds.), *Biochemistry of Mitochondria*, Academic Press, New York, 1967, p. 75.
198   J. B. CHAPPELL, *Brit. Med. Bull.*, 24 (1968) 150.
199   S. PAPA, J. M. TAGER, E. QUAGLIARIELLO AND E. C. SLATER (Eds.), *The Energy Level and Metabolic Control in Mitochondria*, Adriatica, Bari, 1969.
200   G. D. GREVILLE, in J. M. LOWENSTEIN (Ed.), *Citric Acid Cycle. Control and Compartmentation*, Marcel Dekker, New York, 1969, p. 1.
201   J. B. CHAPPEL AND A. R. CROFTS, in J. M. TAGER, S. PAPA, E. QUAGLIARIELLO AND E. C. SLATER (Eds.), *Regulation of Metabolic Processes in Mitochondria, (BBA Library, Vol. 7)*, Amsterdam, 1966, p. 293.
202   J. B. CHAPPELL, *Biochem. J.*, 90 (1964) 225.
203   J. B. CHAPPELL, *Biochem. J.*, 100 (1966) 43P.
204   A. J. MEIJER AND J. M. TAGER, *Biochem. J.*, 100 (1966) 79P.
205   H. W. HELDT, H. JACOBS AND M. KLINGENBERG, *Biochem. Biophys. Res. Commun.*, 18 (1965) 174.
206   M. KLINGENBERG AND E. PFAFF, in J. M. TAGER, S. PAPA, E. QUAGLIARIELLO AND E. C. SLATER (Eds.), *Regulation of Metabolic Processes in Mitochondria, (BBA Library, Vol. 7)*, Elsevier, Amsterdam, 1966, p. 180.
207   M. KLINGENBERG AND E. PFAFF, *Biochem. Soc. Symp. (Cambridge, Engl.)*, 27 (1968) 105.
208   E. PFAFF AND M. KLINGENBERG, *Eur. J. Biochem.*, 6 (1968) 66.
209   M. KLINGENBERG, H. W. HELDT AND E. PFAFF, in S. PAPA, J. M. TAGER, E. QUAGLIARIELLO AND E. C. SLATER (Eds.), *The Energy Level and Metabolic Control in Mitochondria*, Adriatica, Bari, 1969, p. 237.
210   P. V. VIGNAIS AND E. D. DUEE, *Bull. Soc. Chim. Biol.*, 48 (1966) 1169.
211   P. V. VIGNAIS, E. D. DUEE, P. M. VIGNAIS AND J. HUET, *Biochim. Biophys. Acta*, 118 (1966) 465.
212   J. B. CHAPPELL AND B. H. ROBINSON, *Biochem. Soc. Symp. (Cambridge, Engl.)*, 27 (1968) 123.
213   B. H. ROBINSON AND J. B. CHAPPELL, *Biochem. Biophys. Res. Commun.*, 28 (1967) 249.
214   J. M. TAGER, *Biochim. Biophys. Acta*, 73 (1963) 341.
215   E. J. DE HAAN AND J. M. TAGER, *Biochim. Biophys. Acta*, 153 (1968) 98.
216   J. M. TAGER, E. J. DE HAAN AND E. C. SLATER, in J. M. LOWENSTEIN (Ed.), *Citric Acid Cycle. Control and Compartmentation*, Marcel Dekker, New York, 1969, p. 213.
217   S. PAPA, R. D'ALOYA, A. J. MEIJER, J. M. TAGER AND E. QUAGLIARIELLO, in S. PAPA, J. M. TAGER, E. QUAGLIARIELLO AND E. C. SLATER (Eds.), *The Energy Level and Metabolic Control in Mitochondria*, Adriatica, Bari, 169, p. 159.
218   S. M. F. FERGUSON AND G. R. WILLIAMS, *J. Biol. Chem.*, 241 (1966) 3696.
219   A. J. MEIJER, J. M. TAGER AND K. VAN DAM, in S. PAPA, J. M. TAGER, E. QUAGLIARIELLO AND E. C. SLATER (Eds.), *The Energy Level and Metabolic Control in Mitochondria*, Adriatica, Bari, 1969, p. 147.

220 F. PALMIERI AND E. QUAGLIARIELLO, *Abstr. 5th Meeting Federation European Biochem. Soc., Prague, 1968*, p. 133.
221 A. AZZI, J. B. CHAPPELL AND B. H. ROBINSON, *Biochem. Biophys. Res. Commun.*, 29 (1967) 148.
222 D. H. WILLIAMSON, P. LUND AND H. A. KREBS, *Biochem. J.*, 103 (1967) 514.
223 J. M. HASLAM AND H. A. KREBS, *Biochem. J.*, 104 (1967) 51P.
224 D. E. GRIFFITHS AND J. M. HASLAM, *Biochem. J.*, 104 (1967) 52P.
225 B. H. ROBINSON AND J. B. CHAPPELL, *Biochem. J.*, 105 (1967) 18P.
226 C. C. CHILDRESS AND B. SACKTOR, *Science*, 154 (1966) 268.
227 J. L. GAMBLE JR., *J. Biol. Chem.*, 240 (1965) 2668.
228 J. L. GAMBLE JR. AND J. A. MAZUR, *J. Biol. Chem.*, 242 (1967) 67.
229 S. R. MAX AND J. L. PURVIS, *Biochem. Biophys. Res. Commun.*, 21 (1965) 587.
230 E. J. HARRIS, in S. PAPA, J. M. TAGER, E. QUAGLIARIELLO AND E. C. SLATER (Eds.), *The Energy Level and Metabolic Control in Mitochondria*, Adriatica, Bari, 1969, pp. 31 and 135.
231 E. J. HARRIS, *Biochem. J.*, 109 (1968) 247.
232 P. MITCHELL, *Biol. Rev. Cambridge Phil. Soc.*, 41 (1966) 445.
233 W. S. LYNN AND R. H. BROWN, *Arch. Biochem. Biophys.*, 114 (1966) 260.
234 E. J. HARRIS, K. VAN DAM AND B. C. PRESSMAN, *Nature*, 213 (1967) 1126.
235 E. QUAGLIARIELLO AND F. PALMIERI, in S. PAPA, J. M. TAGER, E. QUAGLIARIELLO AND E. C. SLATER (Eds.), *The Energy Level and Metabolic Control in Mitochondria*, Adriatica, Bari, 1969, p. 45.
236 C.MOORE AND B. C. PRESSMAN, *Biochem. Biophys. Res. Commun.*, 15 (1964) 562.
237 J. B. CHAPPELL AND A. R. CROFTS, *Biochem. J.*, 95 (1965) 393.
238 H. A. LARDY, S. N. GRAVEN AND S.ESTRADA-O, *Federation Proc.*, 26 (1967) 1355.
239 S. N. GRAVEN, S. ESTRADA-O AND H. A. LARDY, *Proc. Natl. Acad. Sci. (U.S.)*, 56 (1966) 654.
240 K. VAN DAM AND E. J. HARRIS, *Abstr. 4th Meeting Federation European Biochem. Soc., Oslo, 1967*, p. 12.
241 F. PALMIERI, M. CISTERNINO AND E. QUAGLIARIELLO, *Biochim. Biophys. Acta*, 143 (1967) 625.
242 K. VAN DAM AND E. C. SLATER, *Proc. Natl. Acad. Sci. (U.S.)*, 58 (1967) 2015.
243 E. J. HARRIS, M. P. HÖFER AND B. C. PRESSMAN, *Biochemistry*, 6 (1967) 1348.
244 B. C. PRESSMAN, in S. PAPA, J. M. TAGER, E. QUAGLIARIELLO AND E. C. SLATER (Eds.), *The Energy Level and Metabolic Control in Mitochondria*, Adriatica, Bari, 1969, p. 87.
245 B. C. PRESSMAN, E. J. HARRIS, W. S. JAGGER AND J. H. JOHNSON, *Proc. Natl. Acad. Sci. (U.S.)*, 58 (1967) 1949.
246 B. C. PRESSMAN, in L. ERNSTER AND Z. DRAHOTA (Eds.), *Mitochondria, Structure and Function (FEBS Symp. Vol. 17)*, Academic Press, London, 1969, p. 315.
247 K. VAN DAM AND C. S. TSOU, in S. PAPA, J. M. TAGER, E. QUAGLIARIELLO AND E. C. SLATER (Eds.), *The Energy Level and Metabolic Control in Mitochondria*, Adriatica, Bari, 1969, p. 21.
248 E. C. SLATER, in S. PAPA, J. M. TAGER, E. QUAGLIARIELLO AND E. C. SLATER (Eds.), *The Energy Level and Metabolic Control in Mitochondria*, Adriatica, Bari, 1969, p. 15.

Chapter II

Fatty Acid Metabolism

SALIH J. WAKIL AND EUGENE M. BARNES JR.

Department of Biochemistry, Duke University Medical Center, Durham, N. C. (U.S.A.)

1. Introduction

Fatty acids are present in cells throughout nature and are encountered most commonly in ester linkage to a variety of complex lipids. Fatty acids occur in a spectrum of chain lengths from acetic acid (C_2) to lignoceric acid (C_{24}) and in various isomeric or substituted forms such as saturated, unsaturated, hydroxy, or branched-chain acids. The most prevalent fatty acids have 16 or 18 carbon atoms in their hydrocarbon chain. However, fatty acids of a number of other chain lengths with an even or odd number of carbon atoms are common in many tissues, although they are ordinarily found at comparably much lower levels than the C_{16} and C_{18} acids.

Unsaturated fatty acids are thought to have a particularly important role in the structure and function of cellular lipids. The *cis* configuration of the double bond appears to be ubiquitous for unsaturated fatty acids. In the polyunsaturated acids the olefinic bonds are present in a polyallyl configuration separated from one another by a methylene group. The distribution of unsaturated fatty acids varies from tissue to tissue. Polyunsaturated fatty acids represent a major class of the fatty acids of plant and animal tissues. However, polyunsaturated acids rarely occur in bacteria, which normally contain monounsaturated fatty acids or their cyclopropane derivatives.

This work is a survey of present knowledge concerning fatty acid metabolism and the mechanisms of metabolic control.

[57]

2. Fatty acid oxidation

(a) β-Oxidation of saturated acids

The β-oxidation mechanism for fatty acid degradation was first proposed by Knoop in 1904. This is the pathway for oxidation of fatty acids by successive removal of acetate (C_2) units[1,2]. The sequence of events necessary for β-oxidation are: (*i*) formation of the fatty acyl coenzyme A thioester, (*ii*) α,β-dehydrogenation of the acyl-CoA, (*iii*) hydration of α,β-unsaturated acyl-CoA, (*iv*) oxidation of the β-hydroxyacyl-CoA, and (*v*) thiolytic cleavage of the β-ketoacyl-CoA.

(i) Formation of the coenzyme A thioester

The initial step in β-oxidation is the activation of unesterified fatty acid to the corresponding thioester of CoA. A series of acyl-CoA synthetases catalyze this activation according to the reaction:

$$RCOOH + CoASH + ATP \underset{Mg^{2+}}{\overset{\text{acyl-CoA synthetase}}{\rightleftharpoons}} RCOSCoA + AMP + PP_i$$

Three different acyl-CoA synthetases have been described which vary according to their specificities for the chain length of their fatty acid substrates. The acetyl-CoA synthetase (acetate:CoA ligase (AMP), EC 6.2.1.1) utilizes acetate, propionate, and acrylate in a decreasing order of activity. Webster[3] found a molecular weight of 35 200 for the crystalline acetyl-CoA synthetase from bovine heart mitochondria. This enzyme binds one mole of acetyladenylate per mole and has a multiple requirement for monovalent cations (K^+) and divalent cations (Mg^{2+}) for optimal activity[4,5]. The cations are required for the half-reaction forming the acetyladenylate–enzyme intermediate in acetyl-CoA synthesis as shown (Eqns. 1–3).

$$\text{Acetate} + \text{ATP} + \text{E} \rightleftharpoons \text{E–(acetyladenylate)} + PP_i \qquad (1)$$

$$\text{E–(acetyladenylate)} + \text{CoA} \rightleftharpoons \text{acetyl-CoA} + \text{AMP} + \text{E} \qquad (2)$$

The sum of these two reactions is:

$$\text{Acetate} + \text{ATP} + \text{CoA} \rightleftharpoons \text{acetyl-CoA} + \text{AMP} + PP_i \qquad (3)$$

A second acyl-CoA synthetase (acid:CoA ligase (AMP), EC 6.2.1.2) was isolated from beef-liver mitochondria by Mahler et al.[6]. This enzyme is specific for fatty acids of medium chain length (C_4 to C_{11}) and is also active with 3-hydroxy and 2,3- or 3,4-unsaturated fatty acid substrates. Kornberg and Pricer[7] have described an acyl-CoA synthetase in microsomes which exhibits activity with long-chain fatty acids (C_{10} to C_{20}).

A fatty acid activating enzyme has been isolated from mitochondrial membranes that requires GTP rather than the usual ATP substrate. This enzyme, described by Galzigna et al.[8], produces orthophosphate rather than pyrophosphate in the phosphorolysis reaction. The overall reaction is given below (Eqn. 4). This enzyme utilizes long-chain fatty acids and a phospholipid

$$RCOOH + GTP + CoASH \rightleftharpoons RCOSCoA + GDP + P_i \qquad (4)$$

requirement has been demonstrated[8]. It is sensitive to inhibition by fluoride and orthophosphate.

Transacylation is another mechanism by which acyl-CoA can be synthesized. This reaction is catalyzed by a thiophorase (Eqn. 5). The fatty acid

$$Succinyl\text{-}CoA + RCOOH \rightleftharpoons Succinate + RCOSCoA \qquad (5)$$

utilized is normally a short-chain acid (C_4, C_6) or a corresponding β-keto derivative[9]. This activity is found only in extrahepatic tissues.

(ii) The α,β-dehydrogenation of acyl-CoA

A series of acyl-CoA dehydrogenases catalyze the general desaturation reaction shown below (Eqn. 6). Three such enzymes which differ in their

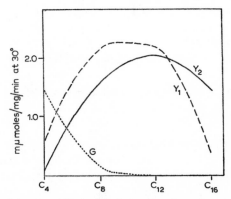

Fig. 1. Specificity of fatty acyl-CoA dehydrogenases for substrates of different chain lengths. G, butyryl-CoA dehydrogenase; Y_1 and Y_2, acyl-CoA dehydrogenases (Crane *et al.*[13]).

chain-length specificities have been isolated from pig liver mitochondria[10-12]. A butyryl-CoA dehydrogenase (butyryl-CoA:(acceptor) oxidoreductase, EC 1.3.99.2) and two acyl-CoA dehydrogenases (acyl-CoA:(acceptor) oxidoreductase, EC 1.3.99.3) were shown to have the relative specificities

$$RCH_2CH_2COSCoA + acceptor \rightarrow$$

$$trans\text{-}RCH = CHCOSCoA + reduced\ acceptor \qquad (6)$$

illustrated in Fig. 1. The spectrum of substrates dehydrogenated by these enzymes insures oxidation of acyl-CoA derivatives of C_4 to C_{20} chain length to the corresponding α,β-unsaturated derivative.

The family of acyl-CoA dehydrogenases are flavoproteins which have the flavin–adenine dinucleotide (FAD) prosthetic group. The abstracted electrons of the substrate are transferred first to the FAD of the dehydrogenase and then to yet another FAD-flavoprotein, the electron-transferring flavoprotein. This latter flavoprotein is in direct linkage to the cytochrome b of the mitochondrial electron transport system[13,14].

(iii) The hydration of α,β-unsaturated fatty acyl-CoA

Through the action of enoyl-CoA hydratase (L-3-hydroxyacyl-CoA hydrolyase, EC 4.2.1.17) the trans-α,β-unsaturated acyl-CoA derivatives arising from the previous reaction are hydrated, thus forming the β-hydroxyacyl-CoA derivatives[15,16]. This reaction is shown in Eqn. 7. The enoyl-CoA

$$trans\text{-}RCH = CHCOSCoA + H_2O \rightleftharpoons L\text{-}RCHOHCH_2COSCoA \qquad (7)$$

hydratase which catalyzes this conversion has a broad substrate specificity and can hydrate both cis- and trans-α,β-unsaturated fatty acyl-CoA esters[17]. The trans isomer is hydrated to the L(+) antipode of β-hydroxyacyl-CoA and the cis derivative is converted to the corresponding D(−) isomer. The mechanism of this stereospecific hydration is shown in Fig. 2. This model was based on the assumptions that a three-point attachment[18] arises between enzyme and substrate, that addition of the elements of water always occurs from the same side (the attack leads to the opening of the lower ["light"] bond, Fig. 2), and further that the same hydrogen of the α-carbon is removed as H_2O in the reverse direction. Similar mechanisms have been proposed for the hydration of fumarate[19], the dehydration of citrate[20], and the oxidation of NAD$^+$ by alcohol dehydrogenase[21].

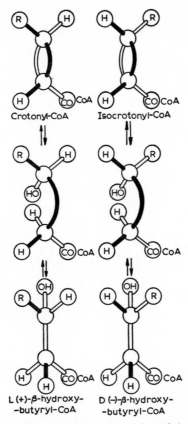

Fig. 2. A three-dimensional diagrammatic representation of the reaction of unsaturated
acyl-CoA hydratase on crotonyl-CoA and isocrotonyl-CoA (Wakil[17]).

(iv) Oxidation of the β-hydroxyacyl-CoA

The L-β-hydroxyacyl-CoA derived from the previous reaction is oxidized
in the presence of NAD^+ and the L-β-hydroxyacyl-CoA dehydrogenase
(L-3-hydroxyacyl-CoA:NAD oxidoreductase, EC 1.1.1.35) to the corresponding β-ketoacyl-CoA ester, as given in Eqn. 8. The L-β-hydroxyacyl-CoA

$$\text{L-RCHOHCH}_2\text{COSCoA} + \text{NAD}^+ \rightleftharpoons \underset{\underset{\text{O}}{\|}}{\text{RCCH}_2}\text{COSCoA} + \text{NADH} + \text{H}^+ \quad (8)$$

dehydrogenase has a strict specificity for the L isomer, but can utilize
hydroxyacyl derivatives of a variety of chain lengths[22,23].

References p. 100

(v) *Thiolytic cleavage of the β-ketoacyl-CoA*

Thiolytic cleavage of β-ketoacyl-CoA is the terminal step in β-oxidation. This reaction which is catalyzed by a thiolase (acyl-CoA:acetyl-CoA *C*-acyltransferase, EC 2.3.1.16) is shown below (Eqn. 9). Crystalline thiolase

$$RCCH_2COSCoA + CoASH \rightleftharpoons RCOSCoA + CH_3COSCoA \qquad (9)$$
$$\underset{O}{\overset{\|}{}}$$

prepared from ox liver[24] has a broad substrate specificity — cleaving β-ketoacyl-CoA derivatives of C_4 to C_{16} chain lengths. The relative activities of these substrates with the thiolase are: $C_4 : C_6 : C_8 : C_{10} : C_{12} : C_{16} =$ 1 : 5.1 : 4.3 : 3.8 : 3.6 : 3.6. An active thiol group of thiolase participates in formation of an acyl-S-enzyme intermediate which is involved in the overall cleavage reaction as shown (Eqns. 10 and 11). The thiolase reaction is

$$RCOCH_2COSCoA + HS\text{-}E \rightarrow RCOS\text{-}E + CH_3COSCoA \qquad (10)$$

$$RCOS\text{-}E + CoA\text{-}SH \rightarrow RCOS\text{-}CoA + HS\text{-}E \qquad (11)$$

reversible but the equilibrium constant greatly favors acetyl-CoA formation from acetoacetyl-CoA $(K = 6 \cdot 10^4)$.

(b) *β-Oxidation of unsaturated fatty acids*

The unsaturated fatty acids occurring in nature are characterized by several common structural features. The double bonds are generally found to be in the *cis* configuration and the olefinic bonds of polyenoic acids are separated by one methylene group. The position of the olefinic bond within the hydrocarbon chain is usually several carbon atoms removed from either the methyl or carboxyl end. A convenient method of classification of unsaturated fatty acids is by the position of the double bond from the ω-CH_3 carbon of the hydrocarbon chain. According to this system the commonly occurring unsaturated acids can be divided into four groups; the palmitoleic, oleic, linoleic, and linolenic series.

The β-oxidation of these unsaturated fatty acids requires at least two enzymatic steps in addition to the scheme for saturated fatty acids discussed above. For example, the oxidation of linoleic acid requires activation to the CoA thioester, followed by oxidation to the α,β-unsaturated derivative, hydration to the β-ketoacyl-CoA, and cleavage to acetyl-CoA and *cis*,

cis-hexadec-7,10-dienoyl-CoA. These reactions are catalyzed by enzymes common to both saturated and unsaturated acid pathways. The sequence is repeated twice more resulting in formation of two additional acetyl-CoA molecules and *cis,,cis*-$\Delta^{3,6}$-C_{12}-CoA. This latter compound is not a substrate for acyl-CoA dehydrogenase or for enoyl-CoA hydratase. However, through the intervention of an isomerase the *cis*-Δ^3 double bond is converted to a *trans*-Δ^2 configuration as shown below (Eqn. 12). This Δ^3-*cis*-Δ^2-*trans*-

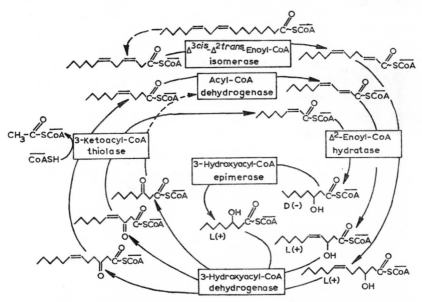

enoyl-CoA isomerase has been isolated from rat-liver mitochondria[25]. The *cis*-Δ^6-*trans*-Δ^2-C_{12}-CoA generated by the isomerase is hydrated by the enoyl-CoA hydratase to the corresponding L-*β*-hydroxyacyl-CoA, which is then oxidized to the *β*-ketoacyl-CoA and cleaved to generate *cis*-Δ^4-decenoyl-

Fig. 3. Sequence of reactions by which unsaturated fatty acids are oxidized to acetyl-CoA (Stoffel and Caesar[27]).

CoA and acetyl-CoA. A subsequent cycle of β-oxidation yields cis-Δ^2-octenoyl-CoA which in turn is hydrated by the enoyl-CoA hydratase. The product of the hydratase reaction is the D-β-hydroxyacyl derivative according to the mechanism already outlined (section 2a, iii, p.60). The D($-$) isomer is epimerized by the action of D($-$)-β-hydroxyacyl-CoA epimerase[25,26] to the L($+$) antipode, which in turn is the substrate for the L($+$)-β-hydroxyacyl-CoA dehydrogenase. As shown in Fig. 3, it is possible to oxidize poly-unsaturated fatty acids via the β-oxidation cycle to acetyl-CoA with the aid of the isomerase and epimerase. All of these enzymes are located in the mitochondria. It has been shown that the rates of oxidation of saturated (palmitic) and polyunsaturated fatty acids are equal in this organelle[27].

(c) The oxidation of odd-chain fatty acids

Many tissues have significant amounts of odd-chain (C_{15} and C_{17}) fatty acids, although the concentration of these acids is generally much less than the even-chain acids. Fatty acids with an odd number of carbon atoms are oxidized via the β-oxidation pathway to acetyl-CoA and one equivalent of propionyl-CoA. Propionyl-CoA can also arise by direct activation of propionic acid by the acetyl-CoA synthetase or from degradation of branched-chain amino acids. The oxidation of propionyl-CoA in animal tissues involves conversion to succinyl-CoA, according to Eqns. 13–15.

Propionyl-CoA carboxylase (propionyl-CoA: carbon dioxide ligase (ADP), EC 6.4.1.3) catalyzes the conversion of propionyl-CoA to methylmalonyl-CoA. Crystalline propionyl-CoA carboxylase[28] has been isolated from pig heart and has a molecular weight of 700 000. The enzyme contains 4 moles

$$*CH_3CH_2COSCoA + HCO_3^- + ATP \rightleftharpoons \underset{\substack{|\\ COOH}}{\overset{\substack{COSCoA\\ |}}{H_3*C-C-H}} + ADP + P_i \quad (13)$$

(S)-Methylmalonyl-CoA

$$\underset{\substack{|\\ COOH}}{\overset{\substack{COSCoA\\ |}}{H_3\overset{*}{C}-C-H}} \rightleftharpoons \underset{\substack{|\\ COSCoA}}{\overset{\substack{COOH\\ |}}{H_3\overset{*}{C}-C-H}} \quad (14)$$

(S)-Methylmalonyl-CoA (R)-Methylmalonyl-CoA

$$
\begin{array}{ccc}
\text{COOH} & & \text{COOH} \\
| & & | \\
\text{H}_3\text{*C--C--H} & \rightleftharpoons & \text{CH}_2 \\
| & & | \\
\text{COSCoA} & & \text{*CH}_2 \\
& & | \\
(R)\text{-Methylmalonyl-CoA} & & \text{COSCoA} \\
& & \text{Succinyl-CoA}
\end{array}
\qquad (15)
$$

of biotin per mole, suggesting 4 subunits of 175 000 molecular weight. The role of biotin in this carboxylase is the same as that observed for other biotin enzymes. The formation of a carboxylated intermediate (carboxybiotin enzyme) is involved in the catalytic process. This intermediate serves as CO_2 donor to propionyl-CoA. (This mechanism is discussed in greater detail in section 3a, p. 66.)

The carboxylase gives rise to methylmalonyl-CoA in the (S)-configuration which is not the proper stereoisomer for utilization by the mutase enzyme[29]. Through the intervention of methylmalonyl-CoA racemase[30], (S)-methylmalonyl-CoA is epimerized to (R)-methylmalonyl-CoA. The methylmalonyl-CoA mutase (methylmalonyl-CoA:CoA-carboxylmutase, EC 5.4.99.2) then converts the (R) isomer to succinyl-CoA[31,32]. The mutase enzyme contains coenzyme B_{12} which is involved in the intramolecular rearrangement of the substrate[33]. During this rearrangement, the CoA-S-CO- unit is transferred to the methyl group[34] as shown in reaction 15. All of these enzymes are also found in the mitochondria.

3. Fatty acid biosynthesis

At the time when the mechanism of β-oxidation of fatty acids was first fully recognized, it was assumed that fatty acid biosynthesis was accomplished by a reversal of the β-oxidation pathway. However, the discovery by Gibson et al.[35] that fatty acid synthesis in avian liver requires ATP and bicarbonate provided the first indication of a difference in the synthetic and degradative pathways. It was observed that the absolute requirement for bicarbonate did not lead to incorporation of bicarbonate carbon into fatty acids and that the required ATP undergoes phosphorolysis to ADP and P_i. The role of bicarbonate was made clear by the experiments of Wakil[36] that established the requirement of bicarbonate for synthesis of malonyl-CoA from acetyl-CoA. Malonyl-CoA is the C_2 donor for elongation of the fatty acid ultimately resulting in palmitate synthesis. The overall reactions involved in synthesis of long-chain fatty acids from acetyl-CoA have been elucidated by several laboratories[37-41]. These may be shown as given in Eqns. 16 and 17. The

$$CH_3COSCoA + HCO_3^- + ATP \rightleftharpoons HOOCCH_2COSCoA + ADP + P_i \quad (16)$$

$$CH_3COSCoA + 7\ HOOCCH_2COSCoA + 14\ NADPH + 14\ H^+ \rightarrow$$
$$CH_3CH_2(CH_2CH_2)_6\ CH_2COOH + 7\ CO_2 + 14\ NADP^+ + 8\ CoA + 6\ H_2O \quad (17)$$

initial step is catalyzed by acetyl-CoA carboxylase which has been shown to have a biotin prosthetic group[42]. The second reaction (Eqn. 17) is catalyzed by a group of enzymes, collectively referred to as fatty acid synthetase. This group of enzymes may exist as a tight multienzyme complex such as those found in animal tissues[37,43] or yeast[44], or in a readily dissociable form such as that found in bacteria[45-47] or in plant tissue[48].

An acyl primer of short chain length is required for the conversion of malonyl-CoA to long-chain fatty acids[49]. This primer becomes the methyl terminus of the fatty acid and malonyl-CoA supplies the remaining carbon atoms of the molecule. Acetyl-CoA is generally the most effective precursor or "primer" but other short straight- or branched-chain acyl derivatives may also be utilized[37,50]. Elongation of propionyl-CoA or isopropionyl-CoA by fatty acid synthesis results in odd-chain or branched-chain fatty acids, respectively.

(a) Acetyl-CoA carboxylase

Acetyl-CoA carboxylase (acetyl-CoA:CO_2 ligase (ADP), EC 6.4.1.2) was the first enzyme to be recognized of the class of biotin enzymes. The protein has a covalently linked biotin necessary for enzymatic activity. The egg white protein, avidin, which binds biotin completely blocks carboxylase activity[42]. Many biotin enzymes have now been isolated and all appear to have the same general mechanism of action. Two steps are required in the carboxylation of acetyl-CoA:

$$\text{Biotin protein} + ATP + HCO_3^- \rightleftharpoons CO_2 \sim \text{biotin protein} + ADP + P_i \quad (18)$$

$$CO_2 \sim \text{biotin protein} + CH_3COSCoA \rightleftharpoons$$
$$\text{biotin protein} + {}^-OOCCH_2COSCoA \quad (19)$$

The sum of these reactions is:

$$ATP + HCO_3^- + CH_3COSCoA \rightleftharpoons ADP + P_i + {}^-OOCCH_2COSCoA \quad (20)$$

Incubation of the biotin enzyme with $H^{14}CO_3^-$ and ATP results in formation of $^{14}CO_2\sim$ biotin enzyme. On incubation of this isolated complex with acetyl-CoA, $^{14}CO_2$ is transferred to acetyl-CoA thus forming malonyl-CoA. The carboxybiotinyl linkage has been shown to be 1'-N-carboxybiotinyl enzyme as shown below. Biotin itself is linked to the protein *via* the ε-amino groups of lysine in analogous fashion to biocytin[51].

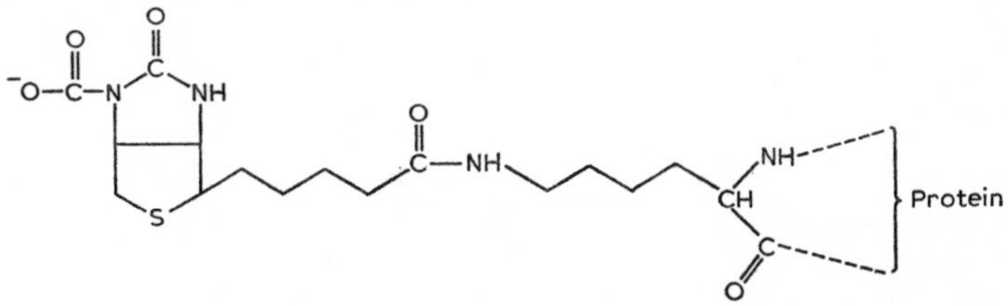

All biotin enzymes appear to give the same structure as shown[52–56]. The mechanism for the formation of the carboxybiotinyl enzyme is not clear, although the findings of Kaziro *et al.*[57] indicate that bicarbonate rather than free carbon dioxide is the precursor in the carboxylation reaction. The carboxylation of biotin may occur by a concerted mechanism as shown in Eqn. 21 or by a stepwise reaction involving a phosphorylated intermediate as illustrated in Eqns. 22 and 23 (ref. 44). The observation of ADP–ATP exchange in the presence of pyruvate carboxylase[58] suggests that the stepwise mechanism is the more likely.

Alberts and Vagelos[59] have recently fractionated the acetyl-CoA carboxylase of *Escherichia coli* into three proteins required for the overall reaction. One of these fractions is a biotin-containing protein of low molecular weight which has no apparent catalytic activity. One of the two remaining proteins is a biotinyl carboxylase which catalyzes the formation of $CO_2\sim$ biotinyl protein (reaction 18); the third protein catalyzes a transcarboxylation from the carboxybiotinyl protein to the acetyl-CoA acceptor (reaction 19). Their findings suggest that one biotinyl protein may be common to the family of carboxylases and that specificity of the enzyme for acceptor may be conferred by the transcarboxylating protein. However, confirmation of this hypothesis must await further experimentation.

The carboxylase-dependent transfer of the carboxyl group from biotin protein to acceptor is stereospecific. The entering carboxyl group retains the same configuration as the departing hydrogen atom[44], as shown in reaction 24. This mechanism would also explain the stereospecific formation of (S)-methylmalonyl-CoA by propionyl-CoA carboxylase[29].

The half-life of the carboxybiotinyl protein complex is about 10 min in the absence of substrate. The complex is rendered more unstable by the presence of substrates or allosteric effectors (citrate or isocitrate) or a combination of the two[60-62]. The free energy of the cleavage of the CO_2-biotinyl protein complex as written in Eqn. 25 has been estimated at -4.7 kcal/mole at

$$CO_2 \sim \text{biotinyl protein} + H^+ \rightarrow CO_2 + \text{biotinyl protein} \qquad (25)$$

pH 7.0 (ref. 56). This value is sufficient to permit carboxylation of acceptors without an additional energy source.

The marked stimulation of fatty acid synthesis in extracts of pigeon liver by citrate and isocitrate can be explained by the ability of these acids to exert positive allosteric control on acetyl-CoA carboxylase. The activity of this enzyme can be stimulated 15 to 16-fold by citrate or isocitrate. The unstimulated carboxylase appears to be the rate-limiting step in fatty acid biosynthesis, while citrate-activated enzyme can produce malonyl-CoA at a rate equal to the conversion of malonyl-CoA to fatty acid by the fatty acid synthetase[63]. The regulation of the synthesis of malonyl-CoA by citrate or isocitrate may be physiologically important in the control of fatty acid synthesis.

Studies of the acetyl-CoA carboxylase from rat adipose and liver tissue and from chicken liver have elucidated the mechanism of citrate stimulation [64–67]. These findings indicate that citrate or isocitrate increase the V_{max} of the carboxylase reaction but do not affect the K_m for substrates. Citrate binds the enzyme with high affinity (dissociation constant $= 2 \cdot 10^{-6}$–$3 \cdot 10^{-6}$) and induces polymerization of enzyme molecules. The association phenomenon has been studied extensively in homogeneous acetyl-CoA carboxylase preparations from chicken liver[67,68]. The polymeric and protomeric forms of the enzyme can be reversibly generated. Polymer formation is promoted by anions (citrate, isocitrate, malonate, tricarballylate, sulfate, and orthophosphate), acetyl-CoA, high protein concentrations, and a pH of 6.0 to 7.0. Dissociation of the polymer to protomer can be effected by Cl^-, a pH above 7.5, and formation of carboxybiotinyl enzyme. Citrate and isocitrate can induce formation of polymeric carboxybiotinyl enzyme, but the same is not true for tricarballylate or P_i. In addition, these latter two compounds do not stimulate enzymatic activity.

The polymeric form of acetyl-CoA carboxylase has a molecular weight of $4 \cdot 10^6$–$8 \cdot 10^6$ and the protomer, 410 000. Each protomeric molecule contains one biotinyl prosthetic group[38,69] and one binding site for acetyl-CoA or citrate. Dodecyl sulfate causes the dissociation of the protomer into subunits with a $s^o_{20,w}$ of 4.3 S having an estimated molecular weight of 110 000. This suggests four subunits per protomer of acetyl-CoA carboxylase. One subunit contains biotin and is converted to the carboxybiotinyl intermediate, while another may be involved in carboxylation of the biotin prosthetic group and carboxyl transfer to acceptor. The other two subunits may be involved in allosteric control of carboxylase and contain sites for binding of malonyl-CoA and acetyl-CoA.

Examinations of acetyl-CoA carboxylase by electron microscopy have indicated a correlation between state of aggregation and level of enzymatic activity[69]. The protomer, shown to be enzymatically inactive, has a minimum dimension of 70–156 Å and a maximum dimension of 100–300 Å. In the presence of isocitrate the active polymeric form is obtained which is composed of 10 to 20 protomer molecules which are assembled in a linear fashion to give filaments 70–100 Å wide and up to 4000 Å long.

(b) Fatty acid synthetases

The second overall step in fatty acid synthesis is the conversion of malonyl-CoA to palmitic acid. This reaction is catalyzed by a complex of enzymes collectively referred to as fatty acid synthetase. The overall conversion of malonyl-CoA to palmitate requires acetyl-CoA and NADPH as shown in reaction 17. The fatty acid synthetase has been isolated as a multienzyme complex in homogeneous form from both animal liver and yeast[37,40,43]. Since the enzyme requires free sulfhydryl groups for activity and since free intermediates do not accumulate during fatty acid synthesis, protein-bound acyl derivatives have been postulated as intermediates in the reaction[40].

The fatty acid synthesizing system of E. coli differs from the animal and yeast complexes since it can be readily dissociated into its component enzymes[45–47]. The acyl intermediates of the E. coli system are bound via a thioester linkage to a low-molecular-weight protein named acyl carrier protein (ACP)[47,70]. The protein has a 4'-phosphopantetheine prosthetic group onto which the intermediates of fatty acid synthesis are bound. The role of ACP in fatty acid biosynthesis is analogous to that of coenzyme A in β-oxidation of fatty acids. The acyl intermediates in both pathways are attached to the thiol group of 4'-phosphopantetheine. In fatty acid synthesis, acetyl and malonyl groups are transferred from the appropriate CoA derivative to ACP before their conversion to fatty acids can occur. All ensuing acyl intermediates in the pathway remain bound to the ACP molecule.

The sequence of reactions necessary for synthesis of fatty acids from acetyl-CoA and malonyl-CoA may be summarized[47,70] in the equations 26–31.

$$CH_3COS\text{-}CoA + ACP\text{-}SH \rightleftharpoons CH_3COS\text{-}ACP + CoA\text{-}SH \qquad (26)$$

$$HOOCCH_2COS\text{-}CoA + ACP\text{-}SH \rightleftharpoons HOOCCH_2COS\text{-}ACP + CoA\text{-}SH \quad (27)$$

$$CH_3COS\text{-}ACP + HOOCCH_2COS\text{-}ACP \rightarrow$$
$$CH_3COCH_2COS\text{-}ACP + CO_2 + ACP\text{-}SH \quad (28)$$

$$CH_3COCH_2COS\text{-}ACP + NADPH + H^+ \rightleftharpoons$$
$$D(-)\text{-}CH_3CHOHCH_2COS\text{-}ACP + NADP^+ \quad (29)$$

$$D(-)\text{-}CH_3CHOHCH_2COS\text{-}ACP \rightleftharpoons CH_3CH\text{=}CHCOS\text{-}ACP + H_2O \quad (30)$$

$$CH_3CH\text{=}CHCOS\text{-}ACP + NADPH + H^+ \rightarrow$$
$$CH_3CH_2CH_2COS\text{-}ACP + NADP^+ \quad (31)$$

The acyl groups of acetyl-CoA and malonyl-CoA are transferred to ACP by their respective transacylase enzymes, the acetyl-CoA–ACP transacylase and malonyl-CoA–ACP transacylase (reactions 26 and 27). Acetyl-ACP and malonyl-ACP are converted to acetoacetyl-ACP by the acyl-malonyl-ACP condensing enzyme (reaction 28). The acetoacetyl-ACP thus produced is subsequently reduced to β-hydroxybutyryl-ACP, dehydrated to crotonyl-ACP, and finally reduced to butyryl-ACP (reactions 29–31). Butyryl-ACP is then free to participate in another condensation step (reaction 28) which results in formation of β-ketohexanoyl-ACP. Reduction of this compound followed by dehydration and another reduction (reactions 29–31) generates hexanoyl-ACP. Five more cycles of this reaction sequence yields palmityl-ACP. The palmityl-ACP product is then hydrolyzed by a specific thioesterase to palmitic acid and ACP, according to reaction 32.

$$CH_3(CH_2)_{14}COS\text{-}ACP + H_2O \rightarrow CH_3(CH_2)_{14}COOH + ACP\text{-}SH \quad (32)$$

In general this sequence of reactions appears to be common to all fatty acid synthesizing systems.

(c) Acyl carrier protein

The acyl-carrier protein (ACP) from *E. coli* has been purified to homogeneity and its chemical structure has been extensively studied[73,74]. The native protein has a sedimentation coefficient ($s^{\circ}_{20,w}$) of 1.34 S and a low frictional coefficient indicating that ACP is a compactly folded, sparingly hydrated globular protein[75]. Native ACP exhibits optical rotatory dispersion properties typical of a globular protein with ordered structure. ACP may be completely and reversibly denatured by 6 M guanidine hydrochloride.

Studies of the structure of ACP have shown that the molecule consists of a single polypeptide chain with serine as the NH_2-terminus and a COOH-terminal alanine. Cysteine and cystine are not present in the protein, but a thiol group is present which is necessary for coenzymatic activity. This thiol

TABLE I

AMINO ACID COMPOSITION OF ACP

Amino acid	Assumed number of residues/molecule
Lysine	4
Histidine	1
Arginine	1
Aspartic acid	9
Threonine	6
Serine	3
Glutamic acid	18
Proline	1
Glycine	4
Alanine	7
Valine	7
Methionine	1
Isoleucine	7
Leucine	5
Tyrosine	1
Phenylalanine	2
β-Alanine[a]	1
Cysteamine[a,b]	1

The total number of residues was 77.
[a] Not included in the totals.
[b] Measured as taurine.

group is the site for acyl intermediate binding and has been shown to be the cysteamine moiety of a 4'-phosphopantetheine prosthetic group. This prosthetic group is linked to the protein *via* a phosphodiester bond to a serine residue of the polypeptide[71,72].

The amino acid composition of ACP from *E. coli* is given in Table I. This composition differs slightly from previous reports[70,76], presumably because

```
        1                                   10
NH₂—Ser—Thr—Ile—Glu—Glu—Arg—Val—Lys—Lys—Ile—Ile—Gly—Glu—
                      20
Gln—Leu—Gly—Val—Lys—Gln—Glu—Glu—Val—Thr—Asp—Asn—Ala—Ser—
            30                         *                    40
Phe—Val—Glu—Asp—Leu—Gly—Ala—Asp—Ser—Leu—Asp—Thr—Val—Glu—
                                  50
Leu—Val—Met—Ala—Leu—Glu—Glu—Glu—Phe—Asp—Thr—Glu—Ile—Pro—
                        60
Asp—Glu—Glu—Ala—Glu—Lys—Ile—Thr—Thr—Val—Gln—Ala—Ala—Ile—
70                      77
Asp—Tyr—Ile—Asn—Gly—His—Gln—Ala—COOH
```

Fig. 4. The complete amino acid sequence of acyl carrier protein from *E. coli*.

of impurities in earlier preparations. The composition shown in Table I corresponds exactly with the complete amino acid sequence of ACP shown in Fig. 4. This sequence was determined by sequential analyses of the various peptides after partial chemical or enzymatic hydrolysis of ACP[73,74].

The sequence of amino acids of ACP given in Fig. 4 has several interesting features. The sequence indicates a molecular weight of 8847 for ACP. The polypeptide has 14 residues of glutamic acid and 7 of aspartic acid, but only 4 residues of glutamine and 2 of asparagine. The isoelectric point is estimated at pH 4.2, a value close to the pH at which ACP is least soluble. The molecule contains but a few basic amino acids which are located mainly near the termini of the polypeptide chain. The acidic amino acids, on the other hand, appear with great frequency throughout the chain. The regions of highest acidity are residues 47–49 and 56–58 where Glu–Glu–Glu and Asp–Glu–Glu are found, respectively. Acidic amino acids occur frequently in the area between residues 47 and 60 where 9 of 14 residues are either aspartic or glutamic acids. The molecule does not appear to have any areas that contain an appreciable number of hydrophobic amino acids, with the possible exception of residues 62–72 which have only one Glu residue. The prosthetic group, 4′-phosphopantetheine, is attached by a phosphodiester linkage to the hydroxyl group of serine 36. This would indicate that the point of attachment of the fatty acyl moieties to ACP occurs near the center of the polypeptide chain.

The observation that ACP appears to be a typical globular protein in solution and consideration of its amino acid sequence have led to the hypothesis that the native molecule has an unusually high density of charged side-chains at the surface. The importance of such surface structure to the coenzymatic function of ACP remains to be elucidated.

The activity of ACP peptides or ACP derivatives in fatty acid synthesis has been examined by Majerus[77]. Removal of the first 6 peptides from the NH$_2$-terminus results in loss of coenzymatic activity. However, acetylation of the molecule or deletion of 3 residues from the carboxyl terminal end with carboxypeptidase A does not result in any loss of activity. Considerably more information is needed to evaluate the role which structure plays in the unique function of ACP.

An enzyme which catalyzes the removal of the prosthetic group from ACP (reaction 33) has been identified in *E. coli* extracts[78]. This ACP hydrolase

$$\text{ACP} \xrightarrow{\text{Mn}^{2+}} \text{apo-ACP} + 4'\text{-phosphopantetheine} \qquad (33)$$

(ACPase) is an ACP-specific phosphodiesterase which requires divalent cations for activity. Enzymatic activity is stimulated by sulfhydryl compounds such as 2-mercaptoethanol or dithiothreitol. At the present time, the role of the ACPase in ACP metabolism is not clear. However, this enzyme may be involved in the control of holo-ACP levels within the cell.

The biosynthesis of ACP has recently been studied by Elovson and Vagelos[79] who isolated a holo-ACP synthetase from extracts of E. coli. This enzyme catalyzes the reversible transfer of 4'-phosphopantetheine from reduced CoA to apo-ACP, according to reaction 34. This enzyme has a high

$$\text{CoA} + \text{apo-ACP} \xrightarrow{\text{Mg}^{2+}} \text{holo-ACP} + 3',5'\text{-adenosine diphosphate} \qquad (34)$$

affinity for apo-ACP ($K_m = 4 \cdot 10^{-7}M$) and is specific for CoA. Oxidized CoA and dephospho-CoA are not substrates for the enzyme. This enzyme may be of importance in regulation of the relative levels of ACP and CoA in the cell. This type of control may be involved in regulating the synthetic and oxidative pathways of fatty acid metabolism.

(d) The enzymes of fatty acid synthesis

(i) Transacylases

The malonyl-CoA–ACP transacylase isolated from E. coli[80,81] catalyzes the specific transfer of the malonate group from CoA to ACP (reaction 27). This enzyme is heat stable and requires a free sulfhydryl group for enzymatic activity. The equilibrium constant for the malonyl transacylase reactions has been estimated at 2.33, indicating a readily reversible reaction.

The acetyl-CoA–ACP transacylase which catalyzes the transfer of short-chain acyl groups from CoA to ACP (reaction 26) has also been isolated from E. coli[80,81]. This reaction is also freely reversible, the equilibrium constant being 2.09. This transacylase is most active with acetyl-CoA as acyl donor, but the enzyme is capable of utilizing propionyl-, butyryl-, hexanoyl- and octanoyl-CoA for transacylation. The rate of transfer decreases with increasing chain length as shown in Table II. The lowered transacylase activity with increasing chain length of substrate parallels the decreased incorporation of these acyl groups of CoA into long-chain fatty acids catalyzed by the fatty acid synthetase system of E. coli (Table II). This finding suggests that incorporation of acyl-CoA derivatives into long-chain fatty acids is limited by the ability of the acyl-CoA–ACP transacylase to convert them to acyl-ACP.

TABLE II

COMPARISON BETWEEN INCORPORATION OF VARIOUS ACYL-CoA ESTERS INTO
FATTY ACIDS BY *E. coli* SYSTEM AND THEIR TRANSACYLATION TO ACP BY
ACETYL TRANSACYLASE

Substrate	Incorporation into fatty acid (%)	Transacylation to ACP (%)
Acetyl-CoA	100[a]	100[a]
Propionyl-CoA	38	23
Butyryl-CoA	26	10
Hexanoyl-CoA	10	5
Octanoyl-CoA	10	10

[a] Arbitrarily taken as 100%. All values are given as percentage of that of acetyl-CoA.

The acetyl transacylase of *E. coli* is a relatively heat-labile enzyme which has an active sulfhydryl group[80]. A [^{14}C]acetyl-S-enzyme intermediate has been isolated by gel filtration on Sephadex G-25 after incubation of the enzyme with [^{14}C]acetyl-CoA. The isolated [^{14}C]acetyl-S-enzyme intermediate has the ability to acylate either CoA or ACP acceptors. These data suggest the following stepwise mechanism for the transacylation reaction (Eqns. 35 and 36).

$$\text{Acetyl-S-CoA} + \text{HS-enzyme} \rightleftharpoons \text{CoASH} + \text{acetyl-S-enzyme} \qquad (35)$$

$$\text{Acetyl-S-enzyme} + \text{ACP-SH} \rightleftharpoons \text{acetyl-S-ACP} + \text{HS-enzyme} \qquad (36)$$

The sum of these reactions is:

$$\text{Acetyl-S-CoA} + \text{ACP-SH} \rightleftharpoons \text{acetyl-S-ACP} + \text{CoA-SH} \qquad (37)$$

(ii) Acyl-malonyl-ACP condensing enzyme

The acyl-malonyl-ACP condensing enzyme[82,83] catalyzes the synthesis of β-ketoacyl-ACP as shown in reaction 38. This enzymatic reaction may be measured in a coupled assay utilizing the β-ketoacyl-ACP reductase as indicated by reactions 38 and 39. Together, these reactions can be expressed as indicated in Eqn. 40. The rate of NADPH oxidation measured by absorption at 340 mμ indicates the rate of the overall reaction described by Eqn. 40.

$$\text{RCOS-ACP} + \text{HOOCCH}_2\text{COS-ACP} \rightarrow$$
$$\text{RCOCH}_2\text{COS-ACP} + \text{ACP} + \text{CO}_2 \qquad (38)$$

$$\text{RCOCH}_2\text{COS-ACP} + \text{NADPH} + \text{H}^+ \rightleftharpoons$$
$$\text{D}(-)\text{-RCHOHCH}_2\text{COS-ACP} + \text{NADP}^+ \quad (39)$$

$$\text{RCOS-ACP} + \text{HOOCCH}_2\text{COS-ACP} + \text{NADPH} + \text{H}^+ \rightarrow$$
$$\text{D}(-)\text{-RCHOHCH}_2\text{COS-ACP} + \text{CO}_2 + \text{ACP} + \text{NADP}^+ \quad (40)$$

The acyl-malonyl-ACP condensing enzyme has an absolute specificity for ACP derivatives and cannot utilize acyl-CoA compounds. The enzyme is markedly inhibited by N-ethylmaleimide and iodoacetamide indicating the involvement of a functional sulfhydryl group in the catalytic process. Since acetyl-ACP protects the enzyme against inhibition by these sulfhydryl blocking reagents, an acyl-S-enzyme intermediate may be involved in the condensation process.

The condensing enzyme can utilize a wide range of chain lengths of acyl-ACP substrates for condensation with malonyl-ACP. Acetyl-, propionyl-, butyryl-, hexanoyl- and octanoyl-ACP are all substrates for condensation, suggesting that the condensing enzyme elongates all the acyl intermediates in the synthesis of palmityl-ACP. The rate of the condensation reaction tends to increase with increasing chain length of the acyl-ACP. This property of the enzyme may be responsible for the observation that acyl-ACP intermediates do not accumulate during fatty acid synthesis.

(iii) β-Ketoacyl-ACP reductase

The β-ketoacyl-ACP reductase catalyzes the NADPH-dependent reduction of β-ketoacyl-ACP (reaction 29). The product of the reaction is the D$(-)$ isomer of β-hydroxyacyl-ACP; this is the optical antipode of the hydroxyacyl-CoA intermediate in β-oxidation. The β-ketoacyl-ACP reductase from E. coli has been purified and studied[81,84]. The E. coli reductase exhibits optimal activity with pH values between 6.0 and 7.0. In this range of pH the reaction strongly favors β-hydroxyacyl-ACP formation; the equilibrium constant at pH 7.0 is $3.9 \cdot 10^7 M$. The enzyme is much more active with ketoacyl-ACP substrates than with the corresponding CoA derivatives. It has a very broad specificity for chain length of the β-ketoacyl-ACP substrate, being equally active on substrates of C_4 to C_{16} chain length[85].

(iv) The β-hydroxyacyl-ACP dehydrases

The conversion of β-hydroxyacyl-ACP thioesters to the corresponding trans-α,β-unsaturated acyl-ACP derivative (reaction 30) is catalyzed by the β-hydroxyacyl-ACP dehydrases. These enzymes are specific for ACP derivatives and cannot utilize CoA thioesters as substrate[86,87]. The dehydrase reaction is freely reversible and is stereospecific since the enzymes have an absolute requirement for the $D(-)$-β-hydroxy compound. The dehydrases are conveniently assayed by a measurement of hydration of α,β-unsaturated acyl-ACP to the appropriate β-hydroxyacyl-ACP *via* coupling to the β-ketoacyl-ACP reductase. This series of reactions is shown below (Eqns. 41 and 42).

$$RCH\!=\!CHCOS\text{-}ACP + H_2O \rightleftharpoons RCHOHCH_2COS\text{-}ACP \qquad (41)$$

$$RCHOHCH_2COS\text{-}ACP + NADP^+ \rightleftharpoons$$
$$RCOCH_2COS\text{-}ACP + NADPH + H^+ \quad (42)$$

The sum of these reactions is:

$$RCH\!=\!CHCOS\text{-}ACP + H_2O + NADP^+ \rightleftharpoons$$
$$RCOCH_2COS\text{-}ACP + NADPH + H^+ \quad (43)$$

The enzyme-dependent formation of β-hydroxyacyl-ACP is measured by the production of NADPH and acetoacetyl-ACP *via* the reductase reaction (Eqn. 42). Acetoacetyl-ACP may be determined with great sensitivity by its absorbance at 303 mμ in the presence of Mg^{2+} at pH 8.5 (Ref. 88).

Three β-hydroxyacyl-ACP dehydrases which differ in their chain length specificities have recently been isolated from *E. coli*[89]. The β-hydroxybutyryl-ACP dehydrase[86] utilizes short-chain β-hydroxyacyl-ACP compounds. This enzyme gives highest rates of hydration with the α,β-unsaturated C_4 derivative ($V_{max}=4100$ mμmoles per min per mg). Enzymatic activity decreases with increasing chain length (V_{max} for $C_6=2300$ mμmoles per min per mg and for $C_8=200$ mμmoles per min per mg) and no activity is observed for 2-decenoyl-ACP. The chain length specificity of this dehydrase is responsible for accumulation of β-hydroxydecanoyl-ACP in the overall synthetic reactions catalyzed by partially resolved fatty acid synthetase of *E. coli*[90]. This same phenomenon has been observed in a synthetase system reconstituted from purified preparations of β-hydroxybutyryl-ACP dehydrase, condensing enzyme, β-ketoacyl-ACP reductase, and enoyl-ACP reductase[91].

The β-hydroxybutyryl-ACP dehydrase has an estimated molecular weight of 26 000. The enzyme is relatively heat stable and has a broad pH optimum (pH 7.5–8.5) for activity. The dehydrase has a free thiol group which is required for enzymatic activity.

References p. 100

The β-hydroxyoctanoyl-ACP dehydrase has been purified over 60-fold from extracts of *E. coli*[89]. The purified enzyme catalyzes the hydration of *trans*-2-enoyl-ACP thioesters of chain lengths C_6, C_8, C_{10}, and C_{12}. The V_{max} values for these substrates are 4, 19, 89, 31, and 41 mμmoles per min per mg, respectively. This dehydrase is unable to utilize C_{14} or C_{16} chain length substrates and is thus specific for 2-enoyl-ACP derivatives of intermediate chain length.

A functional thiol group is also involved in the activity of the β-hydroxyoctanoyl-ACP dehydrase as shown by complete inhibition of activity by 10^{-4} M p-chloromercuribenzoate. This property clearly differentiates the β-hydroxyoctanoyl-ACP dehydrase from the β-hydroxydecanoyl thioester dehydrase described by Kass *et al.*[92] since this latter enzyme is not sensitive to thiol binding reagents.

The β-hydroxypalmityl-ACP dehydrase has been purified over 500-fold from *E. coli*[89]. This enzyme can hydrate 2-dodecenoyl-ACP, 2-tetradecenoyl-ACP, and 2-hexadecenoyl-ACP. The V_{max} values measured for these C_{12}, C_{14}, and C_{16} substrates are 440, 270, and 1330 mμmoles per min per mg of protein, respectively. The lower activity observed with the Δ^2-C_{14}-ACP substrate compared to the C_{12} and C_{16} derivatives may represent the inherent enzyme specificity, although the possibility of a contaminating dehydrase activity has not yet been ruled out.

The range of chain lengths of substrates for the three dehydrases includes the entire chain length spectrum of the intermediates of long-chain fatty acid synthesis, as shown in Fig. 5. The differences in chain length specificities of these dehydrases may be important in the control of fatty acid synthesis in *E. coli*. It has been shown that the limited utilization of β-hydroxyacyl-ACP substrates by the β-hydroxybutyryl-ACP dehydrase is responsible for accumulation of β-hydroxydecanoyl-ACP by a reconstituted fatty acid synthetase[91]. Similarly, the restricted specificities of the β-hydroxyoctanoyl-ACP dehydrase and β-hydroxypalmityl-ACP dehydrase may be involved in synthesis of β-hydroxymyristic acid, a component of cell wall lipids.

(v) The enoyl-ACP reductases

The enoyl-ACP reductase catalyzes the reduction of *trans*-α,β-unsaturated acyl-ACP to the saturated derivative (reaction 31). This activity has been purified 250-fold from extracts of *E. coli*. The reductase reaction is essentially irreversible and one mole of reduced pyridine nucleotide is consumed for each mole of 2-enoyl-ACP reduced. The purified preparations of this reductase are able to utilize either NADPH or NADH as electron donor for reduction of enoyl-ACP substrates.

A comparison of the properties of the NADPH-dependent and NADH-

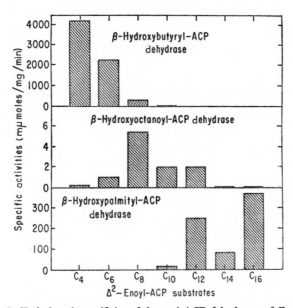

Fig. 5. Chain length specificity of the acyl-ACP dehydrases of *E. coli*.

dependent reductase activity suggests the presence of two distinct enzymes in these preparations, a NADPH–enoyl-ACP reductase and a NADH–enoyl-ACP reductase. The NADPH-dependent activity is unstable on storage at pH 7.5 and has no enzymatic activity observable at pH 8.0. This enzyme has an absolute requirement for ACP thioesters and gives higher rates of reduction with crotonyl-ACP than with longer-chain 2-enoyl-ACP derivatives. The NADPH–enoyl-ACP reuctase is also readily inhibited by *p*-chloromercuribenzoate, iodoacetate, and *N*-ethylmaleimide.

The NADH–enoyl-ACP reductase, on the other hand, is stable to storage at pH 7.5 and has a broad range of pH for optimal enzymatic activity. This enzyme can utilize both enoyl-ACP and enoyl-CoA derivatives of a wide range of chain lengths (C_4 to C_{16}). The NADH-dependent activity is less active with the crotonyl derivative than with the longer-chain-length substrates. This enzyme is not inhibited by *N*-ethylmaleimide treatment which

References p. 100

rather results in a 3-fold stimulation of activity. The NADH–enoyl-ACP reductase is, however, inhibited by iodoacetate and p-hydroxymercuribenzoate.

There does not appear to be a requirement for a flavin prosthetic group in the enoyl-ACP reductases of *E. coli*. The purified enzyme preparation is colorless and trypsin digestion followed by trichloroacetic acid treatment reveals no concealed flavin.

(vi) Palmityl thioesterase

The detailed mechanism for termination of fatty acid biosynthesis at a specific chain length has not been fully elucidated. Fatty acyl-ACP thioesters are the immediate products in bacterial fatty acid synthesizing systems. Palmitate is the principal saturated fatty acid product observed in these systems, although small amounts of myristate and stearate are also produced. The unsaturated fatty acid generated by *E. coli* and certain other bacteria is principally *cis*-vaccenate, but appreciable amounts of palmitoleate are also synthesized. It is not yet clear whether fatty acyl-ACP thioesters are utilized directly, transacylated to CoA, or hydrolyzed to ACP and fatty acids before utilization for complex lipid synthesis.

Two palmityl thioesterases have been recently isolated from *E. coli*[93,167] which catalyze the hydrolysis of long-chain fatty acyl thioesters of ACP and CoA, thus releasing free fatty acid and the respective thiol. Palmityl thioeterase I[93] cleaves thioesters of chain length from C_{12} to C_{18} and acts optimally on palmityl, palmitoleyl, and *cis*-vaccenyl thioesters. Palmityl thioesterase II[167] activity is clearly distinguished from thioesterase I by chromatographic resolution, lack of sensitivity to diisopropyl fluorophosphate, and a broader substrate specificity. Although palmityl thioesterase II also acts optimally on C_{16} esters, it cleaves substrates with chain length less than C_{12} and in addition will hydrolyze β-hydroxyacyl thioesters.

The products of the fatty acid synthetase in the presence of palmityl thioesterase I are unesterified fatty acids. The chain length of the products observed under these conditions is compatible with that expected from specificity of the thioesterase I, suggesting a role for this enzyme in chain termination. However, the acyl-ACP produced by the bacterial fatty acid synthetase may be used directly as the substrate for complex lipid synthesis. It has been shown that both acyl-ACP and acyl-CoA derivatives can serve as donors in the acylation of L-α-glycerol phosphate by preparations from *E. coli*[94,168] and *Clostridium butyricum*[95].

(e) Multienzyme complex of fatty acid synthetase

The fatty acid synthetases of animal tissue and yeast are isolated as tightly associated multienzyme complexes of high molecular weight. All of the components necessary for synthesis of fatty acids from acetyl-CoA, malonyl-CoA, and NADPH (reaction 17) are present in these synthetase complexes. Because of the highly ordered structure and tenacious association of the individual catalytic components of these complexes, the precise mechanism of fatty acid synthesis in these systems is not completely understood. For similar reasons, the high degree of molecular organization has restricted our understanding of structure and function in mitochondria, microsomes, plasma membranes, ribosomes, and other organelles. However, the concepts involved in the mechanism of fatty acid synthesis in *E. coli* have proved to be valuable in application to the synthetase complexes of animals and yeast. In this regard, an ACP-like protein appears to be a component of these complexes and the same basic reactions are required for completion of a fatty acid chain.

(i) The fatty acid synthetase of yeast

Lynen[96] has described the properties of a fatty acid synthetase complex purified 150-fold from yeast cells. The isolated synthetase is homogeneous on ultracentrifugation and yields one component on Tiselius electrophoresis. The molecular weight of the complex is estimated at $2.3 \cdot 10^6$. The enzyme is capable of converting acetyl-CoA and malonyl-CoA to palmityl-CoA or stearyl-CoA according to reaction 44 ($n = 7$ or 8). The product of the overall

$$\text{Acetyl-CoA} + n \text{ malonyl-CoA} + 2n \text{ NADPH} + 2n \text{ H}^+ \rightarrow$$
$$\text{CH}_3(\text{CH}_2\text{CH}_2)_n\text{CO–CoA} + n \text{ CO}_2 + n \text{ CoA} + 2n \text{ NADP}^+ + n \text{ H}_2\text{O} \quad (44)$$

reaction is the fatty acyl-CoA thioester and not free fatty acid as observed in *E. coli* or with the avian liver synthetase[97].

The acyl intermediates in the synthetic process are tightly bound to the complex. Two types of thiol-binding sites are thought to be involved in the operation of the yeast synthetase. A "peripheral" thiol group has been characterized by a marked inhibitory effect of sulfhydryl-binding agents which can be prevented by acetyl-CoA or other acyl-CoA derivatives. This site has been identified as a cysteine residue of the condensing enzyme component of the synthetase[96]. The other thiol site, the "central" sulfhydryl group, is not readily blocked by sulfhydryl-binding reagents and appears to

Priming reaction:

$$CH_3-COSCoA + \overset{HS}{\underset{HS}{\diagup}}Enzyme \rightleftharpoons \overset{HS}{\underset{CH_3-COS}{\diagup}}Enzyme + HSCoA$$

Chain-lengthening reactions:

1)
$$\overset{COOH}{\underset{CH_2-COSCoA}{|}} + CH_3-(CH_2-CH_2)_n-COS\diagdown Enzyme \overset{HS}{} \rightleftharpoons \overset{COOH}{\underset{CH_2-COS}{|}}\diagdown Enzyme + HSCoA$$
$$CH_3-(CH_2-CH_2)_n-COS\diagup$$

2)
$$\overset{COOH}{\underset{CH_2-COS}{|}}\diagdown Enzyme \rightleftharpoons CH_3-(CH_2-CH_2)_n-\overset{O}{\overset{\|}{C}}-CH_2-COS\diagdown Enzyme + CO_2$$
$$CH_3-(CH_2-CH_2)_n-COS\diagup \qquad\qquad HS\diagup$$

3)
$$CH_3-(CH_2-CH_2)_n-\overset{O}{\overset{\|}{C}}-CH_2-COS\diagdown Enzyme + NADPH + H^+ \rightleftharpoons CH_3-(CH_2-CH_2)_n-\overset{OH}{\overset{|}{CH}}-CH_2-COS\diagdown Enzyme + NADP^+$$
$$HS\diagup \qquad\qquad\qquad HS\diagup$$

4)
$$CH_3-(CH_2-CH_2)_n-\overset{OH}{\overset{|}{CH}}-CH_2-COS\diagdown Enzyme \rightleftharpoons CH_3-(CH_2-CH_2)_n-CH=CH-COS\diagdown Enzyme + H_2O$$
$$HS\diagup \qquad\qquad\qquad HS\diagup$$

5)
$$CH_3-(CH_2-CH_2)_n-CH=CH-COS\diagdown Enzyme + NADPH + H^+ \xrightarrow{(FMN)} CH_3-(CH_2-CH_2)_{n+1}-COS\diagdown Enzyme + NADP^+$$
$$HS\diagup \qquad\qquad\qquad HS\diagup$$

6)
$$CH_3-(CH_2-CH_2)_{n+1}-COS\diagdown Enzyme \rightleftharpoons \overset{HS}{\diagdown}Enzyme$$
$$HS\diagup \qquad CH_3-(CH_2-CH_2)_{n+1}-COS\diagup$$

Terminal reaction:

$$CH_3-(CH_2-CH_2)_{n+1}-COS\diagdown Enzyme + HSCoA \rightleftharpoons \overset{HS}{\diagdown}Enzyme + CH_3-(CH_2-CH_2)_{n+1}-COSCoA$$
$$HS\diagup \qquad\qquad\qquad HS\diagup$$

Fig. 6. The mechanism of fatty acid synthesis. The heavy –SH represents the central sulfhydryl group and the light –SH represents the peripheral sulfhydryl group (Lynen, 1967). FMN, flavin mononucleotide coenzyme.

be the thiol group of 4′-phosphopantetheine. This compound is the prosthetic group of the ACP component of the complex, being attached by a phosphodiester linkage to the hydroxyl group of a serine residue in a fashion analogous to *E. coli* ACP (ref. 96).

The involvement of non-thiol sites in the catalytic activity of the yeast synthetase has also been established. These non-thiol groups have a role in the transfer of the acetyl and malonyl groups from their respective CoA thioesters to the "central" sulfhydryl group. These sites have been identified as the hydroxyl groups of active serine residues. These active serine sites are presumably residues of the transacylase components of the multienzyme complex.

The mechanism of adding C_2 units to the growing fatty acid chain requires reactions similar to those described for the *E. coli* system with the exception that a flavin mononucleotide (FMN) coenzyme is involved in the enoyl reductase reaction. The sequence of reactions catalyzed by the yeast synthetase is shown in Fig. 6.

The first step in the biosynthetic scheme is an acetyl group transfer from acetyl-CoA to the "peripheral" sulfhydryl group *via* the intermediate discussed above. This reaction is followed by a malonyl group transfer from malonyl-CoA to the "central" thiol group. The acetyl group is then condensed with the α-carbon of the malonyl-S-enzyme intermediate to form acetoacetyl-S-enzyme and CO_2. The β-ketoacyl intermediate is then subjected to the stepwise reduction shown in Fig. 6 which yields the saturated intermediate. The saturated acyl group is subsequently transferred from the "central" to the "peripheral" thiol group. Another malonyl group is transferred to the "central" sulfhydryl group and a new reaction cycle begins. Repetition of this process occurs until the palmityl- or stearyl-S-enzyme intermediate arises. At this point the fatty acyl group is transferred from the "central" sulfhydryl group to coenzyme A. This terminal reaction accounts for the CoA thioester product observed.

At least 7 individual enzymes, each being responsible for a single reactive step in fatty acid synthesis, appear to be components of the yeast synthetase. The native complex of $2.3 \cdot 10^6$ molecular weight is presumed to contain 3 such complete sets. Electron photomicrographs of negatively stained synthetase preparations show a homogeneous field of oval-shaped particles with a 250-Å longitudinal diameter and 210-Å cross-diameter[44,96].

(ii) The fatty acid synthetase of avian liver

Highly purified preparations of the fatty acid synthetase of pigeon liver have been the subject of extensive study[37,38,43,97−100]. The synthetase preparations appear to be homogeneous by the criteria of electrophoresis and ultracentrifugation and have a molecular weight estimated at 450 000 (or one-fifth the size of the yeast complex). The pigeon liver synthetase can be dissociated into enzymatically inactive subunits which have a molecular weight half that of the intact complex. This dissociation can be effected by incubation of the enzyme with carboxymethyl disulfide or aging in the absence of a reducing agent. Reassociation of the subunits can be accomplished by treatment with dithiothreitol and is accompanied by a recovery of the enzymatic activity[100].

Since the pigeon liver synthetase complex contains one mole of 4'-phosphopantetheine per mole of enzyme, an ACP-like component is thought to be a part of the complex. The reactions involved in the synthesis of palmitate from acetyl-CoA and malonyl-CoA appear to be essentially the same as those described for the yeast system. However, the pigeon liver synthetase differs in the terminal reaction since free palmitate is the product. In addition, the enoyl reductase reaction in the pigeon liver system does not involve flavin[37,43].

The synthetase of pigeon liver can be dissociated into a minimum of 8 different peptides by incubation with 8 M urea, 6 M guanidine–HCl, or phenol–acetic acid–urea. It has not yet been possible to regenerate any of the enzymatic activities after these treatments. This is presumably due to an irreversible denaturation of the individual enzyme components. However, treatment of the complex with 0.5 M guanidine hydrochloride allows chromatographic resolution of the acetyl- and malonyl-transacylase activities from the bulk of the synthetase protein[169].

The properties of the binding sites for acetyl and malonyl groups on the pigeon liver fatty acid synthetase have been recently examined in detail[169,170]. Performic acid oxidation of [14C]acetyl- and [14C]malonyl-labeled synthetase isolated from incubations with the respective CoA thioester has revealed the presence of both thiol and non-thiol acyl-binding sites. Studies on radioactive peptides from these acyl synthetases have demonstrated two thiol-binding sites. One of these sites is the sulfhydryl of the 4'-phosphopantetheine moiety which binds either acetyl or malonyl groups as thioesters. The second thiol site has been identified as a cysteine residue which binds only acetyl groups. The cysteine-thiol site may be differentiated from the other acyl-binding sites by its sensitivity to iodoacetamide and current evidence indicates this site as part of the condensing enzyme component[170]. Acetyl and malonyl groups are also bound to a non-thiol site required for synthetase function; this site has been tentatively identified as the hydroxyl of a serine residue.

Incubation of the pigeon synthetase with high concentrations of N-ethylmaleimide blocks binding of acetyl and malonyl groups at all sites, while low N-ethylmaleimide levels block only the two thiol sites. Iodoacetamide, on the other hand, inhibits binding only at the single cysteine-thiol. From these studies, the order of acetyl binding to the synthetase appears to be first at the non-thiol site with subsequent transfer to 4'-phosphopantetheine thiol and then cysteine sulfhydryl. Malonyl binding follows the same order, except the final transfer to the cysteine site does not occur. A similar sequence of events has also been proposed for the yeast fatty acid synthetase[171].

The reactions now known to be catalyzed by the pigeon liver fatty acid synthetase have been summarized in terms of a model shown in Fig. 7. The

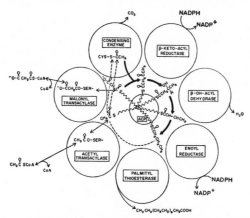

Fig. 7. Schematic representation of the reactions of the pigeon liver fatty acid synthetase complex.

transacylation of acetyl groups from CoA to the 4'-phosphopantetheine moiety (ACP) of the synthetase is mediated by an intermediate acetylation of a non-thiol (serine hydroxyl) binding site. Subsequently, the acetyl group is transferred to the cysteine sulfhydryl of the condensing enzyme. A malonyl group then may be transacylated to the 4'-phosphopantetheine site also through the participation of the non-thiol site. The incoming malonyl group may drive acetyl transfer to the cysteine site because of its higher affinity. The condensation reaction between acetyl and malonyl groups then yields the acetoacetyl derivative which is attached (*via* thioester linkage) at the 4'-phosphopantetheine site. The acetoacetyl derivative is converted to the butyryl thioester by the usual reduction, dehydration, and second reduction steps and finally transferred to the cysteine site. Then the addition on another C_2 unit is initiated by transacylation of a second malonyl group to the 4'-phosphopantetheine site, and the cycle is repeated. In this manner a C_{16} or C_{18} saturated fatty acyl chain would be synthesized. The terminal reaction is cleavage of this long-chain fatty acyl thioester from the 4'-phosphopantetheine by the participation of palmityl thioesterase. Barnes and Wakil[93] have demonstrated the presence of this activity in the pigeon liver synthetase complex and found that the thioesterase has strict specifity for C_{16} and C_{18} thioesters. The final reaction yields the free fatty acid product and generates the unesterified 4'-phosphopantetheine site. This overall model is similar in many respects with that proposed by Lynen[171].

4. Elongation of fatty acids

The major product of the fatty acid synthetases is palmitic acid. The fatty acids of greater chain length are synthesized in the cell by addition of "C_2 units" in stepwise fashion to acids of shorter chain length. Palmitate (C_{16}) may be elongated by such a mechanism of C_2 addition to lignoceric acid (C_{24}).

TABLE III

THE SITES AND COMPONENTS OF FATTY ACID METABOLISM IN ANIMAL TISSUES

System	Cellular localization	Substrates	Pyridine nucleotides	Products
De novo synthesis	Cytosol	Acetyl-CoA+malonyl-CoA	NADPH	Palmitic acid (C_1
Elongation (A)	Microsomes	C_nCoA + malonyl-CoA		$C_n + 2$
		ΔC_nCoA + malonyl-CoA	NADPH	$\Delta C_n + 2$
Elongation (B)	Mitochondria	C_nCoA + acetyl-CoA	NADPH + NADH	$C_n + 2$
		ΔC_nCoA + acetyl-CoA		$\Delta C_n + 2$
Desaturation	Microsomes	C_nCoA	NADH	$\Delta^{11}C_n$
		$\Delta^{11}C_nCoA$	NADH	$\Delta^{7,11}C_n$
α-Oxidation	Microsomes	C_n	—	C_{n-1}
ω-Oxidation	Microsomes	C_9–C_{12}	NADPH	C_9–C_{12}
			NAD+	dicarboxylic aci
β-Oxidation	Mitochondria	$C_{2n}CoA$	NAD+	nC_2CoA

Animal tissues have two different pathways for elongation of fatty acids —one microsomal and one mitochondrial system. The intracellular localization of the various enzyme systems involved in fatty acid metabolism is shown in Table III. The fatty acid synthetase and the acetyl-CoA carboxylase are located in the cytosol, perhaps in an associated form[35]. The mitochondria contain an elongation system which utilizes acetyl-CoA and also the enzymes for β-oxidation of fatty acids. Microsomes have a fatty acid elongating system that requires malonyl-CoA, as well as the α- and ω-oxidation systems.

(*a*) *Microsomal system for elongation*

Microsomes are able to convert fatty acyl-CoA derivatives to longer-chain acids in the presence of malonyl-CoA and NADPH[101–103]. Acetyl-CoA cannot supply carbon for elongation in this system. NADH can serve as electron donor in the microsomal system, but NADPH is a much more effective substrate. Saturated fatty acyl-CoA esters of chain lengths C_{10} to C_{16} are elongated at higher rates than derivatives of other chain lengths. Unsaturated fatty acyl-CoA thioesters are also substrates for this system and are elongated at rates higher than the saturated compounds of comparable chain length. The activity of the microsomal elongation system increases with an increasing number of double bonds in the fatty acyl substrate. This observation leads to the suggestion that the microsomal system is involved in the synthesis of long-chain polyunsaturated acids, such as arachidonate ($C_{20:4}$).

The mechanism of fatty acid elongation by the microsomes has not yet been fully elucidated. However, the best available evidence suggests the elongating process may involve the steps of Eqns. 45–48.

$$RCOSCoA + HOOCCH_2COSCoA \rightarrow$$
$$RCOCH_2COSCoA + CoASH + CO_2 \quad (45)$$

$$RCOCH_2COSCoA + NADPH \rightleftharpoons RCHOHCH_2COSCoA + NADP^+ \quad (46)$$

$$RCHOHCH_2COSCoA \rightleftharpoons RCH=CHCOSCoA + H_2O \quad (47)$$

$$RCH=CHCOSCoA + NADPH \rightarrow RCH_2CH_2COSCoA + NADP^+ \quad (48)$$

(*b*) *Mitochondrial system for elongation*

An enzyme system which is capable of elongation of fatty acids is also present in the mitochondria. In this system, acetyl-CoA is the C_2 donor and both NADH and NADPH are required[38]. The mitochondrial system can add C_2 units to fatty acids of chain lengths C_{10} to C_{22} at the rates given in Fig. 8. Unsaturated fatty acids are also more active C_2 acceptors than their saturated homologues[105,106]. The mechanism of elongation in this system appears to be a reversed β-oxidation pathway, except that the acyl dehydrogenase of β-oxidation is replaced by an enzyme which catalyzes the NADPH-dependent reduction of *trans*-α,β-unsaturated acyl-CoA. This latter enzyme has been called the enoyl-CoA reductase[107,108]. The series

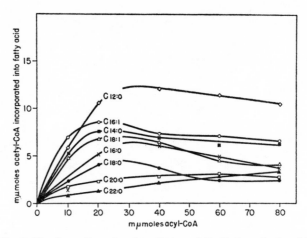

Fig. 8. The elongation of various fatty acyl-CoA's by mitochondria.

of reactions thought to be required for mitochondrial fatty acid elongation is given in reactions 49–52.

$$RCOSCoA + CH_3COSCoA \rightleftharpoons RCOCH_2COSCoA + CoASH \qquad (49)$$

$$RCOCH_2COSCoA + NADH + H^+ \rightleftharpoons RCHOHCH_2COSCoA + NAD^+ \qquad (50)$$

$$RCHOHCH_2COSCoA \rightleftharpoons RCH=CHCOSCoA + H_2O \qquad (51)$$

$$RCH=CHCOSCoA + NADPH + H^+ \rightarrow RCH_2CH_2COSCoA + NADP^+ \qquad (52)$$

5. Desaturation of fatty acids

A saturated fatty acid may be directly converted to the corresponding unsaturated acid by a reaction dependent on reduced pyridine nucleotide and molecular oxygen[109]. This desaturation reaction is catalyzed by an enzyme system localized in the microsomal fraction of animal cells[110,111]. If stearyl-CoA is used as substrate for the desaturase system, oleate (presumably still in CoA thioester linkage) is the product. This system can utilize either NADH or NADPH as an electron donor, but NADH is more effective[112,113]. Cytochrome b_5 and a cyanide-sensitive factor are thought to be components of the desaturase system, but recent evidence indicates that cytochrome P_{450} is not involved[104,112,114]. A functional relationship appears to exist between the microsomal NADH–cytochrome c reductase and the fatty acid desaturating activity[113].

A lipid requirement has been demonstrated for the desaturase system of microsomes[113]. Extraction of microsomes with aqueous acetone results in a loss of desaturase activity which can be restored by addition of micelles of a mixture of phospholipids, triglycerides, and fatty acids. This reconstituted system appears to give essentially the same properties as the native microsomes. The role of lipids in the desaturation system has not yet been established. The lipids may afford a non-aqueous environment for the enzyme system which is required for the reaction. Another possibility is that the lipids may act as an acceptor for the stearyl group from stearyl-CoA, stearyl lipid then being the substrate for desaturation to oleyl lipid[115]. Both acyl-CoA and acyl-phospholipid have been proposed as the immediate substrates for the desaturase system of microsomes[115,116]. However, available evidence does not yet indicate the exact nature of the substrate.

Microsomes also have the capacity to desaturate monoenoic acids to dienoic acids[117]. Oleyl-CoA can be converted to 6,9-octadecadienoic acid in the presence of O_2, reduced pyridine nucleotide, and microsomes. It has not yet been determined if the enzyme system responsible for this conversion is the same as that involved in oleate production.

Microsomes also have the capacity to synthesize poly-unsaturated acids such as arachidonate or eicosatrienoic acids by elongation and desaturation of the proper acyl precursor[118]. The reactions involved in the synthesis of arachidonic acid by such a system are shown in Fig. 9.

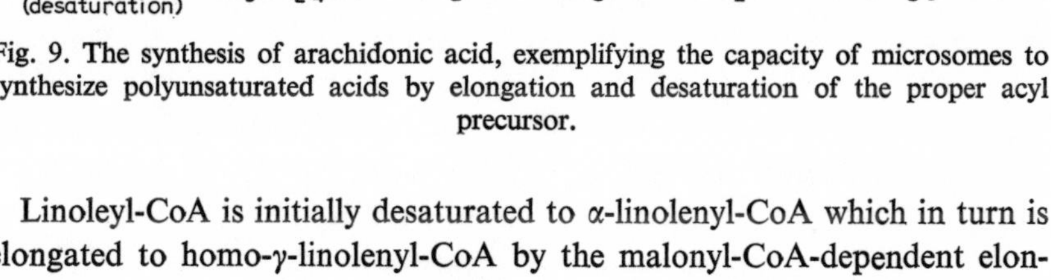

Fig. 9. The synthesis of arachidonic acid, exemplifying the capacity of microsomes to synthesize polyunsaturated acids by elongation and desaturation of the proper acyl precursor.

Linoleyl-CoA is initially desaturated to α-linolenyl-CoA which in turn is elongated to homo-γ-linolenyl-CoA by the malonyl-CoA-dependent elongation system of the microsomes. The homo-γ-linolenyl-CoA thus produced is subjected to a further desaturation to arachidonic acid. This sequence of reactions reveals the cooperative action of the microsomal elongation and desaturation system which can result in synthesis of longer-chain poly-unsaturated fatty acids.

Palmitic acid is the precursor in the synthesis of both saturated and unsaturated fatty acids in animal tissues as shown in Fig. 10. Palmitate can be elongated to long-chain saturated fatty acids (C_{18}, C_{20}, C_{22} and C_{24}); or it can be desaturated to palmitoleic acid ($\Delta^9 C_{16:1}$) and then elongated to produce cis-vaccenic acid ($\Delta^{11} C_{18:1}$) which in turn may be further desat-

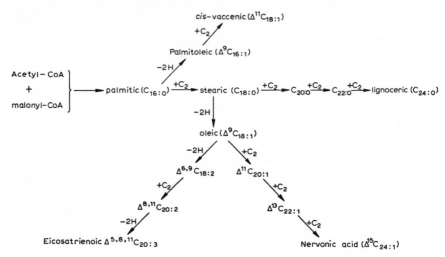

Fig. 10. Biosynthesis of some fatty acids from palmitic acid by animal tissues.

urated, elongated, and desaturated again to generate eicosatrienoic acid ($\Delta^{5,8,11} C_{20:3}$). Oleic acid itself may be subjected to a series of C_2 elongations which can result in nervonic acid ($\Delta^{15} C_{24:1}$).

The fatty acids of the diet can be modified by the pathways discussed so that a variety of polyunsaturated fatty acids of different chain lengths can be synthesized. However, animal tissues do not have the capacity to synthesize linoleic acid and thus must depend on a dietary supply of this essential fatty acid. Once linoleate becomes available for utilization, it may be converted via the desaturation and elongation systems to arachidonic acid and the longer-chain polyunsaturated fatty acids. These compounds are the precursors for synthesis of the newly discovered hormones, the prostaglandins[120,121].

6. α-Oxidation of fatty acids

An enzyme system is present in microsomes which catalyzes the 2-hydroxylation of long-chain fatty acids[122,123]. As a result of this oxidative reaction, decarboxylation of the α-hydroxy fatty acid usually occurs resulting in the formation of fatty acids with an odd number of carbon atoms. The odd-chain acids and α-hydroxy acids are most often found in the cerebroside fraction of brain lipids. The mechanism of this α-oxidation system remains unknown.

7. ω-Oxidation of fatty acids

Another oxidative pathway in fatty acid metabolism involves conversion of the acid to the ω-hydroxy compound which may then be oxidized further to dicarboxylic acids[124]. The enzyme system required for this process is associated with the microsomes and is primarily active on fatty acids of intermediate (C_9 to C_{12}) chain length, although long-chain acids can be utilized[125]. A requirement for molecular oxygen and NADPH has been demonstrated for this system[126]. The ω-oxidation system requires the participation of the microsomal electron transport system, possibly the P_{450} and NADPH–cytochrome c reductase components[127-129]. The details of the mechanism of ω-oxidation have not been completely elucidated, but a NAD^+-dependent oxidation of the ω-hydroxy fatty acid to the dicarboxylic acid appears to be involved.

8. Ketone body formation

The acetyl-CoA which arises by oxidation of fatty acids or of pyruvate is oxidized to CO_2 and H_2O by the citric acid cycle under normal conditions. However, in the metabolic state arising from starvation or diabetes, significant amounts of acetyl-CoA are converted to acetoacetate. The sequence of reactions necessary for the production of acetoacetate involve a β-hydroxy-β-methylglutaryl-CoA intermediate[130], as shown in Eqns. 53–55.

$$2\ CH_3COSCoA \rightleftharpoons CH_3COCH_2COSCoA + CoASH \qquad (53)$$

$$CH_3COCH_2COSCoA + CH_3COSCoA \rightarrow$$

$$\begin{array}{c} CH_3 \\ | \\ HOOCCH_2\!-\!\overset{}{C}\!-\!CH_2COSCoA + CoASH \\ | \\ OH \end{array} \qquad (54)$$

$$
\begin{array}{c}
CH_3 \\
| \\
HOOCCH_2\text{-}C\text{-}CH_2COSCoA + H_2O \rightarrow \\
| \\
OH
\end{array}
$$

$$CH_3COCH_2COOH + CH_3COSCoA \qquad (55)$$

The sum of reactions 53 to 55 is:

$$2\ CH_3COSCoA + H_2O \rightarrow CH_3COCH_2COOH + 2\ CoASH \qquad (56)$$

This pathway serves to regenerate CoA which is needed for increased oxidation of fatty acids under fasting or diabetic conditions. Since the CoA liberated by reaction 56 is utilized immediately in fatty acid activation and oxidation, acetoacetate formation from acetyl-CoA is greatly favored. In a normal metabolic state, citrate synthesis from acetyl-CoA and oxaloacetate provides the source of CoA. However, oxaloacetate is largely consumed by gluconeogenesis in starvation or diabetes and thus restricts the CoA supply *via* the citrate pathway. The increased requirement for CoA brought about by high rates of fatty acid oxidation under these conditions is met by release of CoA from acetyl-CoA by the acetoacetate pathway.

The acetoacetate which arises by this mechanism may be converted to β-hydroxybutyrate. These metabolites may be excreted in the urine or oxidized to CO_2 and H_2O by extrahepatic tissues.

It has been suggested that acetoacetate could arise by a hydrolytic cleavage of acetoacetyl-CoA[131,132] catalyzed by a deacylase. However, attempts to isolate such an enzyme have not been successful and more recent findings indicate that the β-hydroxy,β-methylglutaryl-CoA pathway is the only source of acetoacetate[133,134].

9. Control of fatty acid biosynthesis

The state of present knowledge concerning the mechanism of fatty acid biosynthesis has made possible some investigations into the aspects of control of this synthetic process. However, before discussing this subject, an analysis of the interrelation of several pertinent metabolic pathways is important.

The fatty acid synthetase and the acetyl-CoA carboxylase are located in the cytosol of the cell. The two enzyme systems are associated and may be separated from the supernatant fraction of broken cells by centrifugation at $140\ 000 \times g$ for 2 to 4 h[135]. There is very little information concerning the factors affecting this association.

Dietary carbohydrates supply the principal portion of the "raw materials" needed for synthesis of long-chain fatty acids. Glucose is broken down *via* the glycolytic pathway to pyruvate which is then oxidized by the mitochondrial pyruvate oxidase to acetyl-CoA. Acetyl-CoA is condensed with oxaloacetate to form citrate which then diffuses out of the mitochondrial space. Citrate, in turn, is cleaved by an extramitochondrial enzyme to oxaloacetate and acetyl-CoA[136], according to reaction 57. The acetyl-CoA

Citrate + CoASH + ATP →

$$\text{acetyl-CoA} + \text{oxaloacetate} + \text{ADP} + \text{P}_i \qquad (57)$$

which arises from this pathway is subsequently used for fatty acid synthesis as the acyl primer and as the source of C_2 units for elongation after conversion to malonyl-CoA (reactions 16 and 17)[137,138].

The reductive power for fatty acid synthesis is supplied by NADPH generated by the oxidation of glucose 6-phosphate or the NADH arising from glycolysis. In this latter case, the oxaloacetate produced from citrate cleavage is reduced to malate by NADH. Malate then undergoes oxidative decarboxylation to pyruvate and NADPH[139,140] (Eqns. 58 and 59).

$$\text{Oxaloacetate} + \text{NADH} + \text{H}^+ \xrightleftharpoons{\text{malate dehydrogenase}} \text{malate} + \text{NAD}^+ \qquad (58)$$

$$\text{Malate} + \text{NADP}^+ \xrightarrow{\text{malic enzyme}} \text{pyruvate} + \text{CO}_2 + \text{NADPH} + \text{H}^+ \qquad (59)$$

The sum of reactions 58 and 59 is:

Oxaloacetate + NADH + NADP$^+$ →

$$\text{pyruvate} + \text{CO}_2 + \text{NADPH} + \text{NAD}^+ \qquad (60)$$

The generation of NADPH in either case is closely linked to glucose oxidation. The carbon and hydrogen of fatty acids are thus essentially derived from glucose. It is evident, then, that fatty acid synthesis is dependent on the availability of glucose and the glycolytic activity of the cell.

The strong influence which the nutritional state of the animal has over fatty acid biosynthesis has been recognized for some time. The level of fatty acid synthesis is severely depressed during starvation or diabetes[141,142]. Under these conditions, glucose metabolism is markedly reduced, and thus fatty acid synthesis is impaired. The anabolic activity of the fatty acid synthesizing system is subject to allosteric control by glucose metabolites and to control of enzyme levels *via* protein synthesis.

(a) Regulation of fatty acid synthesis by metabolites

The enzymatic activities of the acetyl-CoA carboxylase and the fatty acid synthetase appear to be modified by the presence of a variety of metabolites. The acetyl-CoA carboxylase catalyzes the first committed step in fatty acid biosynthesis. Under the proper conditions the carboxylase reaction generating malonyl-CoA is also the rate-limiting step in fatty acid synthesis[143]. The activity of this enzyme is markedly stimulated by tricarboxylic acid metabolites[64,144-146]; citrate or isocitrate activate the carboxylase 15 to 16-fold. These metabolites are bound to the acetyl-CoA carboxylase and cause polymerization of the enzyme molecules (see section 3a, p. 66). The concentrations of citrate necessary to produce activation of the carboxylase ($K_m = 6.5 \cdot 10^{-3} M$) are higher than the apparent intracellular concentration of this metabolite, an observation which places the physiological role of the stimulation observed *in vitro* in some doubt.

Citrate does, however, increase the activity of fatty acid synthesis in extracts of liver or lactating mammary gland[137,146,147]. In these systems, citrate affords stimulation not only to acetyl-CoA carboxylase but also provides acetyl-CoA for fatty acid synthesis *via* the cleavage enzyme (reaction 57). It should be noted that the acetate carbons of acetyl-CoA derived from citrate cleavage are the same carbons of acetyl-CoA that originally arose by mitochondrial synthesis of citrate. Thus, citrate is the intermediate between pyruvate and the acetyl-CoA used for synthesis of fatty acids. When rat liver tissue slices are incubated with citrate, fatty acid synthesis is increased and cholesterol synthesis is depressed[148], indicating that the effect of citrate is exercised at the carboxylase step.

The acetyl-CoA carboxylase may also be regulated by feedback control in the form of inhibition by long-chain acyl-CoA derivatives. The inhibition caused by acyl-CoA is competitive with citrate but is non-competitive with respect to the acetyl-CoA, bicarbonate, or ATP substrates[149]. Unesterified fatty acids do not inhibit carboxylase at the concentrations for which fatty acyl-CoA esters are effective. The detergent properties of these acyl-CoA compounds have raised some doubt as to the significance of the carboxylase inhibition[150]. However, the inhibitory concentrations of fatty acyl-CoA observed *in vitro* are comparable to the intracellular levels of these compounds[151]. In addition, the levels of fatty acyl-CoA increase in the metabolic states induced by starvation, diabetes, and high fat intake. Thus, negative feedback control exercised by these compounds may be a factor in regulation of fatty acid biosynthesis.

The rate of fatty acid synthesis in slices and in total extracts of liver tissue from rats in a variety of metabolic states has been examined[152-154]. The rate of fatty acid synthesis in liver slices taken from rats after a 24-h fast was only 1 % of the normal level, while acetyl-CoA carboxylase was 50 % of normal. In tissues from animals fasted for longer periods, however, the activity of the carboxylase is sufficiently low to account for the observed depression of fatty acid synthesis. In addition, the level of citrate in liver tissue from fasted animals is not reduced to a degree consistent with the decrease in fatty acid synthesis[66]. These observations suggest the participation of other mechanisms involved in the control of fatty acid synthesis.

Recently, evidence has been presented which suggests that the fatty acid synthetase complex is itself subject to metabolite control[155]. At concentrations above 10 μM, malonyl-CoA inhibits the enzymatic activity of the pigeon liver fatty acid synthetase complex, increasing the K_m for NADPH by 19-fold. The inhibitory effect of malonyl-CoA may be reduced by NADPH or fructose 1,6-diphosphate. The NADPH effect is competitive with malonyl-CoA; fructose 1,6-diphosphate exerts its effect by a reduction of the K_m for NADPH and an increase in the V_{max} of the reaction. An allosteric mechanism appears to be involved in the malonyl-CoA inhibition *via* a regulatory site (or sites) on the enzyme complex which is distinct from the catalytic sites. The fructose 1,6-diphosphate appears to relieve the malonyl-CoA inhibition either by competition for the regulatory site or binding at a separate site which results in an enzyme form insensitive to malonyl-CoA inhibition. Glucose 1-phosphate and glucose 6-phosphate have an effect similar to that of fructose 1,6-diphosphate, but only at relatively higher concentrations.

The inhibition of the fatty acid synthetase by malonyl-CoA and its reversal by NADPH or fructose 1,6-diphosphate is an attractive control mechanism since it affords a scheme for linking rates of fatty acid synthesis directly to the oxidation of glucose. This scheme also provides a mechanism for regulation of fatty acid synthesis by the immediate precursors involved. Under conditions where NADPH levels are declining, malonyl-CoA consumption *via* the fatty acid synthetase would also decline, and thus malonyl-CoA levels would tend to increase. This would further depress the activity of the fatty acid synthetase. Excess accumulation of malonyl-CoA would be prevented since this metabolite acts as a potent inhibitor of its own synthesis *via* competitive inhibition of the citrate activation of acetyl-CoA carboxylase[69]. Thus the observed malonyl-CoA inhibition of the synthetase and carboxylase may be important in the regulation of fatty acid synthesis during

References p. 100

the initial stages of starvation or diabetes. This aspect of control may be particularly important since citrate levels in liver are not markedly reduced under these conditions[66].

The relationship of fatty acid synthesis to the other key metabolic pathways, *i. e.* glycolysis, gluconeogenesis, and the citric acid cycle, is depicted in Fig. 11. Under normal metabolic conditions with an abundant supply of glucose, glycolysis proceeds at high rates resulting in generation of pyruvate.

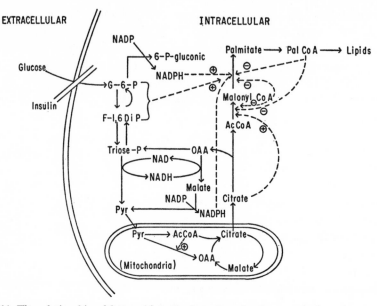

Fig. 11. The relationship of fatty acid synthesis to the other key metabolic pathways, *i.e.* glycolysis, gluconeogenesis, and the citric acid cycle.

Pyruvate enters the mitochondria and is oxidized to acetyl-CoA and carboxylated to form oxaloacetate. These latter two metabolites are condensed to citrate which then leaves the mitochondria and is converted back to acetyl-CoA and oxaloacetate. By the action of the citrate-activated acetyl-CoA carboxylase, acetyl-CoA is converted to malonyl-CoA. This latter compound is rapidly utilized for palmitate synthesis in the presence of NADPH. The source of NADPH is the glycolytic pathway (reactions 58–60) or the pentose cycle. Under these conditions, levels of phosphorylated sugars are high, and the malonyl-CoA inhibition of the fatty acid synthetase is consequently overcome. This circumstance allows continuous conversion of malonyl-CoA to fatty acid. The oxaloacetate arising from citrate cleavage may be reduced to malate which subsequently may be converted to pyruvate or be returned to the mitochondria for utilization in citrate synthesis.

In the metabolic state induced by starvation, when glucose is not in abundant supply, or by diabetes, when glucose transport across the cell membrane is impaired, glycolysis is severely curtailed. The mobilization and oxidation of fatty acids markedly increases, as does gluconeogenesis. The pyruvate which is derived from amino acid degradation is converted to oxaloacetate in the mitochondria. The oxaloacetate may be reduced to malate which leaves the mitochondria. Alternately, oxaloacetate may be condensed with acetyl-CoA to form citrate, although this process occurs at lower rates than normal. Citrate may be oxidized by the tricarboxylic acid cycle or may diffuse trom the mitochondria where it may accumulate at low but appreciable levels. Citrate may be cleaved to yield oxaloacetate which is utilized for gluconeogenesis and acetyl-CoA which is converted to malonyl-CoA. Malonyl-CoA accumulates since it is not actively used for fatty acid synthesis owing to reduced levels of NADPH. The accumulation of malonyl-CoA causes a further decrease in the level of fatty acid synthesis. The increasing level of malonyl-CoA also acts to decrease its own synthesis by inhibition of acetyl-CoA carboxylase. In addition, the increased levels of long-chain fatty acyl-CoA derivatives owing to fatty acid mobilization may exert further inhibitory effects on the acetyl-CoA carboxylase and fatty acid synthetase.

This rather complex situation leads to a finely controlled winding down of fatty acid synthesis. The administration of insulin to diabetic animals or feeding of carbohydrates to starved animals results in a reversal of the above effects and a return to normal levels of fatty acid synthesis.

(b) Regulation of fatty acid synthesis by enzyme synthesis

The mechanisms of control exerted by metabolites discussed above afford the cell a rapid response to changes in nutrient supply. The production of enzymes *via* protein synthesis provides a regulatory response to changes of longer duration. During prolonged starvation or diabetes a decrease in the specific activities of both acetyl-CoA carboxylase and fatty acid synthetase has been observed[145,156−160]. Insulin treatment of diabetic animals or refeeding of starved animals results in a return of the activities of both enzymes to normal levels. The injection of puromycin or actinomycin at the time of refeeding prevents the rise of fatty acid synthesis activities[159]. This observation suggests that the observed changes in specific activities of the enzymes are due to enzyme synthesis. These inhibitors of protein synthesis also block the increases in fatty acid synthesis in response to insulin treatment of diabetic animals[161]. Furthermore, quantitative measurements of acetyl-CoA carboxylase by the use of immunological techniques have shown that the observed changes in specific activity of this enzyme under these conditions are due to changes in the amount of enzyme protein in the cell[162].

It seems clear that the cell is able to control the amounts of the enzymes necessary for fatty acid synthesis in response to metabolic requirements. The mechanism involved in the exercise of this control is not yet known. It has been suggested that fatty acids or their acyl-CoA derivatives are responsible for repression of the synthesis of one or more of the necessary enzymes. This hypothesis is based on the finding that refeeding fasted animals with a high-fat diet fails to induce the production of the fatty acid biosynthetic enzymes, whereas a refeeding with a carbohydrate-rich diet results in maximum synthesis of these enzymes[154,159].

An examination of the control of fatty acid biosynthesis in *Lactobacillus plantarum* has revealed that addition of unsaturated fatty acids to the growth medium results in a marked reduction of the synthesis of fatty acids in this organism[163,164]. This observation is thought to be due to repression of the synthesis of acetyl-CoA carboxylase and the enzymes of the fatty acid synthetase.

A regulatory mechanism which controls the composition of saturated *versus* unsaturated fatty acids in *E. coli* has been studied. The effect of exogenous unsaturated fatty acids on the fatty acid composition of phospholipids was examined in unsaturated fatty acid auxotrophs[172,173]. When each member of a structurally homologous series of *cis*-unsaturated fatty acids served as a growth factor, the percentage of unsaturated fatty acid present in phospholipids increased with increasing chain length or decreasing number of double bonds in the apolar side chain of the supplement. Utilization of exogenous *cis*-unsaturated fatty acids at decreasing growth temperatures between 42° and 27° resulted in increasing amounts of unsaturated fatty acids in phospholipids with decreasing temperature. These observations suggest the operation of a regulatory mechanism that is responsible for maintaining the physical properties of membrane lipids within narrow limits[173]. However, the level at which such control is mediated is not apparent at the present time.

10. Control of fatty acid oxidation

Recently a considerable amount of information has become available concerning the mechanisms involved in the control of fatty acid oxidation. The regulation of this process by metabolite levels has been discussed in detail earlier in this series (Volume 18, Chapter VIII). Our understanding of the control of fatty acid oxidation as exercised by enzyme synthesis rests mainly on studies with *Escherichia coli*[165,166]. This bacterium is able to utilize fatty acids as the sole carbon source for growth only after a lag phase, suggesting that the enzymes of β-oxidation are inducible. Cells which have been grown on fatty acids for several generations are able to oxidize fatty acids at rates considerably higher than amino acid- or glucose-grown cells. The activities of the individual enzymes of β-oxidation are considerably higher in cells whose growth was supported by fatty acids than in those grown on other carbon sources. Since the individual enzymes are induced to the same extent, it appears that the system is under unit control.

It also appears that the ability of fatty acids to induce the β-oxidation system is dependent on their chain length. Long-chain fatty acids such as myristate, palmitate, or oleate are capable of supporting normal growth of the organism, while short-chain acids (C_4 to C_{12}) fail to support growth. It is of interest that these short-chain acids are nevertheless oxidized by resting cells. It has been suggested that the failure of short-chain acids in supporting growth is due to the inability of these acids to induce the enzymes of β-oxidation.

An interaction of long-chain fatty acyl-CoA derivatives with a specific repressor of enzyme expression may be necessary for induction of the β-oxidation system. Mutants of *E. coli* which are deficient in the acyl-CoA synthetase do not have an inducible system of β-oxidation; the specific activity of the other oxidative enzymes remains at the uninduced level regardless of the growth conditions. It seems clear that more information is required, particularly with regard to animal systems, before the significance of this type of regulatory mechanism can be fully appreciated.

REFERENCES

1 D. E. Green, *Biol. Rev. Cambridge Phil. Soc.*, 29 (1954) 330.
2 F. Lynen, *Harvey Lectures Ser.*, 48 (1952–1953) 210.
3 L. T. Webster Jr., *J. Biol. Chem.*, 240 (1965) 4158.
4 L. T. Webster Jr., *J. Biol. Chem.*, 240 (1965) 4164.
5 L. T. Webster Jr., *J. Biol. Chem.*, 241 (1966) 5504.
6 H. M. Mahler, S. J. Wakil and R. M. Bock, *J. Biol. Chem.*, 204 (1953) 453.
7 A. Kornberg and W. E. Pricer Jr., *J. Biol. Chem.*, 204 (1953) 329.
8 L. Galzigna, C. R. Rossi, L. Sartorelli and D. M. Gibson, *J. Biol. Chem.*, 242 (1967) 2111.
9 J. R. Stern, M. J. Coon, A. Del Campillo and M. C. Schneider, *J. Biol. Chem.*, 221 (1956) 15.
10 F. L. Crane, S. Mii, J. G. Hauge, D. E. Green and H. Beinert, *J. Biol. Chem.*, 218 (1956) 701.
11 F. L. Crane and H. Beinert, *J. Biol. Chem.*, 218 (1956) 717.
12 J. G. Hauge, F. L. Crane and H. Beinert, *J. Biol. Chem.*, 219 (1956) 727.
13 F. L. Crane, J. G. Hauge and H. Beinert, *Biochim. Biophys. Acta*, 17 (1955) 293.
14 P. B. Garland, B. Chance, L. Ernester, C. Lee and D. Wong, *Proc. Natl. Acad. Sci. (U. S.)*, 58 (1967) 1696.
15 S. J. Wakil and H. R. Mahler, *J. Biol. Chem.*, 207 (1954) 125.
16 J. R. Stern and A. Del Campillo, *J. Biol. Chem.*, 218 (1956) 985.
17 S. J. Wakil, *Biochim. Biophys. Acta*, 19 (1956) 497.
18 A. G. Ogston, *Nature*, 162 (1948) 963.
19 H. A. Krebs, *Harvey Lectures Ser.*, 44 (1948) 165.
20 V. R. Potter and C. Heidelberger, *Nature*, 164 (1949) 180.
21 H. R. Fischer, E. E. Conn, B. Vennesland and F. H. Westheimer, *J. Biol. Chem.*, 202 (1953) 687.
22 S. J. Wakil, D. E. Green, S. Mii and H. R. Mahler, *J. Biol. Chem.*, 207 (1954) 631.
23 J. R. Stern, *Biochim. Biophys. Acta*, 26 (1957) 448.
24 W. Seubert, I. Lamberts, R. Kramer and B. Ohly, *Biochim. Biophys. Acta*, 164 (1968) 498.
25 W. Stoffel, R. Ditzer and H. Caesar, *Z. Physiol. Chem.*, 339 (1964) 167.
26 J. R. Stern, A. Del Campillo and A. L. Leheringer, *J. Am. Chem. Soc.*, 77 (1955) 1073.
27 W. Stoffel and H. G. Scheefer, *Z. Physiol. Chem.*, 341 (1965) 84; W. Stoffel and H. Caesar, *Z. Physiol. Chem.*, 341 (1965) 76.
28 Y. Kaziro, S. Ochoa, R. C. Warner and J. Y. Chen, *J. Biol. Chem.*, 236 (1961) 1917.
29 M. Specher, M. J. Clark and D. B. Sprinson, *J. Biol. Chem.*, 241 (1966) 872.
30 R. Mazumder, T. Sasakawa, Y. Kaziro and S. Ochoa, *J. Biol. Chem.*, 237 (1962) 3065.
31 P. Lengyel, R. Mazumder and S. Ochoa, *Proc. Natl. Acad. Sci. (U.S.)*, 46 (1960) 1312.
32 R. Mazumder, T. Sasakawa and S. Ochoa, *J. Biol. Chem.*, 238 (1963) 50.
33 R. W. Kellermeyer and H. G. Wood, *Biochemistry*, 1 (1962) 1124.
34 H. Eggerer, P. Overath, F. Lynen and E. R. Stadtman, *J. Am. Chem. Soc.*, 82 (1960) 2643.
35 D. M. Gibson, E. B. Titchener and S. J. Wakil, *J. Am. Chem. Soc.*, 80 (1958) 2908.
36 S. J. Wakil, *J. Am. Chem. Soc.*, 80 (1958) 6465.
37 R. Bressler and S. J. Wakil, *J. Biol. Chem.*, 236 (1961) 1643.

38 S. J. WAKIL, *J. Lipid Res.*, 2 (1961) 1.
39 S. J. WAKIL, *Ann. Rev. Biochem.*, 32 (1963) 369.
40 F. LYNEN, *Federation Proc.*, 20 (1961) 941.
41 P. R. VAGELOS, *Ann. Rev. Biochem.*, 33 (1964) 139.
42 S. J. WAKIL AND D. M. GIBSON, *Biochim. Biophys. Acta*, 41 (1960) 122.
43 R. Y. HSU, G. WASSON AND J. W. PORTER, *J. Biol. Chem.*, 240 (1965) 3736.
44 F. LYNEN, *Biochem. J.*, 102 (1967) 381.
45 A. W. ALBERTS, P. GOLDMAN AND P. R. VAGELOS, *J. Biol. Chem.*, 238 (1963) 557.
46 W. J. LENNARZ, R. J. LIGHT AND K. BLOCH, *Proc. Natl. Acad. Sci. (U.S.)*, 48 (1962) 840.
47 S. J. WAKIL, E. L. PUGH AND F. SAUER, *Proc. Natl. Acad. Sci. (U.S.)*, 52 (1964) 106.
48 R. D. SIMONI, R. S. CRIDDLE AND P. K. STUMPF, *J. Biol. Chem.*, 242 (1967) 573.
49 S. J. WAKIL AND J. GANGULY, *J. Am. Chem. Soc.*, 81 (1959) 2597.
50 M. G. HORNING, D. B. MARTIN, A. KARMEN AND P. R. VAGELOS, *J. Biol. Chem.*, 236 (1961) 669.
51 L. D. WRIGHT, E. L. CRESSON, H. R. SKEGGS, T. R. WOOD, R. L. PECK, D. E. WOLF AND K. FOLKERS, *J. Am. Chem. Soc.*, 74 (1952) 1996.
52 S. NUMA, E. RINGELMANN AND F. LYNEN, *Biochem. Z.*, 340 (1964) 228.
53 M. WAITE AND S. J. WAKIL, *J. Biol. Chem.*, 241 (1966) 1909.
54 M. D. LANE AND F. LYNEN, *Proc. Natl. Acad. Sci. (U.S.)*, 49 (1963) 379.
55 M. C. SCRUTTON, D. B. KEECH AND M. F. UTTER, *J. Biol. Chem.*, 240 (1965) 574.
56 H. G. WOOD, H. LOCHMILLER, C. RIEPERFINGER AND F. LYNEN, *Biochem. Z.*, 337 (1963) 247.
57 Y. KAZIRO, L. F. HASS, P. D. BOYER AND S. OCHOA, *J. Biol. Chem.*, 237 (1962) 1460.
58 M. C. SCRUTTON AND M. F. UTTER, *J. Biol. Chem.*, 240 (1965) 3714.
59 A. W. ALBERTS AND P. R. VAGELOS, *Proc. Natl. Acad. Sci. (U.S.)*, 59 (1968) 561.
60 Y. KAZIRO AND S. OCHOA, *J. Biol. Chem.*, 236 (1961) 3131.
61 J. KNAPPE, B. WENGER AND U. WIEGAND, *Biochem. Z.*, 337 (1963) 232.
62 E. RYDER, C. GREGOLIN, H. C. CHANG AND M. D. LANE, *Proc. Natl. Acad. Sci. (U.S.)*, 57 (1967) 1455.
63 H. C. CHANG, I. SERDMAN, G. TECHOR AND M. D. LANE, *Biochem. Biophys. Res. Commun.*, 28 (1967) 682.
64 D. B. MARTIN AND P. R. VAGELOS, *J. Biol. Chem.*, 237 (1962) 1787.
65 P. R. VAGELOS, A. W. ALBERTS AND D. B. MARTIN, *J. Biol. Chem.*, 238 (1963) 533.
66 F. LYNEN, M. MATSUHASHI, S. NUMA AND E. SCHWEIZER, in J. K. GRANT (Ed.), *The Control of Lipid Metabolism, Biochem. Soc. Symp. No. 24*, Academic Press, New York, 1964, p. 43.
67 C. GREGOLIN, E. RYDER AND M. D. LANE, *J. Biol. Chem.*, 243 (1968) 4227.
68 C. GREGOLIN, E. RYDER, R. C. WARNER, A. K. KLEINSCHMIDT, H. C. CHANG AND M. D. LANE, *J. Biol. Chem.*, 243 (1968) 4236.
69 C. GREGOLIN, E. RYDER, A. K. KLEINSCHMIDT, R. C. WARNER AND M. D. LANE, *Proc. Natl. Acad. Sci. (U.S.)*, 56 (1966) 1751.
70 P. W. MAJERUS, A. W. ALBERTS AND P. R. VAGELOS, *Proc. Natl. Acad. Sci. (U.S.)*, 51 (1964) 1231.
71 E. L. PUGH AND S. J. WAKIL, *J. Biol. Chem.*, 240 (1965) 4727.
72 P. W. MAJERUS, A. W. ALBERTS AND P. R. VAGELOS, *J. Biol. Chem.*, 240 (1965) 4723.
73 T. C. VANAMAN, S. J. WAKIL AND R. L. HILL, *J. Biol. Chem.*, 243 (1968) 6409.
74 T. C. VANAMAN, S. J. WAKIL AND R. L. HILL, *J. Biol. Chem.*, 243 (1968) 6420.
75 T. TAKAGI AND C. TANFORD, *J. Biol. Chem.*, 243 (1968) 6432.
76 F. SAUER, E. L. PUGH, S. J. WAKIL, R. DELANEY AND R. L. HILL, *Proc. Natl. Acad. Sci. (U.S.)*, 52 (1964) 1360.

77 P. W. MAJERUS, Science, 159 (1968) 428.
78 P. R. VAGELOS AND A. R. LARABEE, J. Biol. Chem., 242 (1967) 1776.
79 J. ELOVSON AND P. R. VAGELOS, J. Biol. Chem., 243 (1968) 3603.
80 I. P. WILLIAMSON AND S. J. WAKIL, J. Biol. Chem., 241 (1966) 2326.
81 A. W. ALBERTS, P. W. MAJERUS, B. TALAMO AND P. R. VAGELOS, Biochemistry, 3 (1964) 1563.
82 A. W. ALBERTS, P. W. MAJERUS AND P. R. VAGELOS, Biochemistry, 4 (1965) 2265.
83 R. E. TOOMEY AND S. J. WAKIL, J. Biol. Chem., 241 (1966) 1159.
84 R. E. TOOMEY AND S. J. WAKIL, Biochim. Biophys. Acta, 116 (1966) 189.
85 S. J. WAKIL, M. MIZUGAKI, M. SHAPIRO AND G. WEEKS, in L. BOLIS AND B. A. PETHICA (Eds.), Membrane Models and the Formation of Biological Membranes, North Holland, Amsterdam, 1968, p. 122.
86 M. MIZUGAKI, G. WEEKS, R. E. TOOMEY AND S. J. WAKIL, J. Biol. Chem., 243 (1968) 3661.
87 P. W. MAJERUS, A. W. ALBERTS AND P. R. VAGELOS, J. Biol. Chem., 240 (1965) 618.
88 J. R. STERN, M. J. COON AND A. DEL CAMPILLO, J. Am. Chem. Soc., 75 (1952) 1517.
89 M. MIZUGAKI, A. C. SWINDELL AND S. J. WAKIL, Biochem. Biophys. Res. Commun., 33 (1968) 520.
90 E. L. PUGH, F. SAUER, M. WAITE, R. E. TOOMEY AND S. J. WAKIL, J. Biol. Chem., 241 (1966) 2635.
91 G. WEEKS AND S. J. WAKIL, J. Biol. Chem., 243 (1968) 1180.
92 L. R. KASS, D. J. H. BROCK AND K. BLOCH, J. Biol. Chem., 242 (1967) 4418.
93 E. M. BARNES JR. AND S. J. WAKIL, J. Biol. Chem., 243 (1968) 2955.
94 G. P. AILHAUD, P. R. VAGELOS AND H. GOLDFINE, J. Biol. Chem., 242 (1967) 4459.
95 H. GOLDFINE, G. P. AILHAUD AND P. R. VAGELOS, J. Biol. Chem., 242 (1967) 4466.
96 F. LYNEN, in H. J. VOGEL, J. O. LAMPEN AND V. BRYSON (Eds.), Organizational Biosynthesis, Academic Press, New York, 1967, p. 243.
97 R. BRESSLER AND S. J. WAKIL, J. Biol. Chem., 237 (1962) 1441.
98 I. P. WILLIAMSON, J. K. GOLDMAN AND S. J. WAKIL, Federation Proc., 25 (1966) 340.
99 P. C. YANG, P. H. BUTTERWORTH, R. M. BOCK AND J. W. PORTER, J. Biol. Chem., 242 (1967) 3501.
100 P. H. BUTTERWORTH, P. C. YANG, R. M. BOCK AND J. W. PORTER, J. Biol. Chem., 242 (1967) 3508.
101 W. STOFFEL AND K. L. ACH, Z. Physiol. Chem., 337 (1964) 123.
102 D. H. NUGTEREN, Biochim. Biophys. Acta, 106 (1965) 280.
103 H. MOHRHAUER, K. CHRISTIANSEN, M. V. GAN, M. DEUBIG AND R. T. HOLMAN, J. Biol. Chem., 242 (1967) 4507.
104 S. J. WAKIL, in R. M. C. DAWSON AND D. M. RHODES (Eds.), Metabolism and Physiological Significance of Lipids, John Wiley and Sons, Ltd., New York, 1964, p.3.
105 S. C. BOONE, Doctoral dissertation, Duke University, 1964.
106 W. R. HARLAN JR. AND S. J. WAKIL, J. Biol. Chem., 238 (1963) 3216.
107 G. R. LANGDON, J. Am. Chem. Soc., 77 (1955) 5190.
108 W. SEUBERT, I. LAMBERTS, R. KRAMER AND B. OHLY, Biochim. Biophys. Acta, 164 (1968) 498.
109 D. K. BLOOMFIELD AND K. BLOCH, J. Biol. Chem., 235 (1960) 337.
110 K. BERNARD, J. VON BÜLOW-KÖSTER AND H. WAGNER, Helv. Chim. Acta, 42 (1959) 152.
111 J. B. MARSH AND A. T. JAMES, Biochim. Biophys. Acta, 60 (1962) 320.
112 N. OSHINO, Y. IMAI AND R. SATO, Biochim. Biophys. Acta, 128 (1966) 13.
113 P. D. JONES, P. W. HOLLOWAY, R. O. PELUFFO AND S. J. WAKIL, J. Biol. Chem., 244 (1969) 744.

114 N. Oshino, Y. Imai and R. Sato, *Abstr. IV, 7th Intern. Congr. Biochem.*, Tokyo, *1967*, E-20, p. 725.
115 M. I. Gurr, M. P. Robinson and A. T. James, *European J. Biochem.*, 9 (1969) 70.
116 J. Nagai and K. Bloch, *J. Biol. Chem.*, 240 (1965) PC 3702.
117 P. W. Holloway, R. O. Peluffo and S. J. Wakil, *Biochem. Biophys. Res. Commun.*, 12 (1963) 300.
118 J. F. Mead, *Federation Proc.*, 20 (1961) 952.
119 P. W. Holloway and S. J. Wakil, *J. Biol. Chem.*, 239 (1964) 2489.
120 D. A. van Dorp, R. K. Beerthuis, D. H. Nugteren and H. Von Keman, *Biochim. Biophys. Acta*, 90 (1964) 204.
121 S. Bergström, H. Danielsson and B. Samuelsson, *Biochim. Biophys. Acta*, 90 (1964) 207.
122 A. J. Fulco and J. F. Mead, *J. Biol. Chem.*, 236 (1961) 2416.
123 A. J. Fulco, *J. Biol. Chem.*, 242 (1967) 3608.
124 P. E. Verkade, *Chem. Ind. (London)*, 57 (1938) 704.
125 B. Preiss and K. Bloch, *J. Biol. Chem.*, 239 (1964) 85.
126 K. Wakagayashi and N. Shimazono, *Biochim. Biophys. Acta*, 70 (1963) 132.
127 Y. H. Lu and M. J. Coon, *J. Biol. Chem.*, 243 (1968) 1331.
128 M. L. Das, S. Orrenius and L. Ernster, *Eur. J. Biochem.*, 4 (1968) 519.
129 F. Wada, H. Shibata, M. Goto and Y. Sakamoto, *Biochim. Biophys. Acta*, 162 (1968) 518.
130 F. Lynen, U. Henning, C. Bublitz, B. Sorbo and L. Kroplin-Rueff, *Biochem. Z.*, 330 (1958) 269.
131 J. R. Stern, G. L. Drummond, M. J. Coon and A. Del Campillo, *J. Biol. Chem.*, 253 (1960) 313.
132 G. I. Drummond and J. R. Stern, *J. Biol. Chem.*, 253 (1960) 318.
133 I. A. Caldwell and G. I. Drummond, *J. Biol. Chem.*, 238 (1963) 64.
134 F. Sauer and J. D. Erfle, *J. Biol. Chem.*, 241 (1966) 30.
135 D. M. Gibson, E. B. Titchener and S. J. Wakil, *Biochim. Biophys. Acta*, 30 (1958) 376.
136 P. A. Srere and F. Lipmann, *J. Am. Chem. Soc.*, 75 (1953) 4874.
137 A. Bhaduri and P. Srere, *Biochim. Biophys. Acta*, 70 (1963) 221.
138 J. M. Lowenstein, in J. K. Grant (Ed.), *The Control of Lipid Metabolism*, Biochem. Soc. Symp. No. 24, Academic Press, New York, 1964, p. 57.
139 H. A. Lardy, V. Paetkau and P. Walter, *Proc. Natl. Acad. Sci. (U.S.)*, 53 (1965) 1410.
140 M. S. Kornacker and E. G. Ball, *Proc. Natl. Acad. Sci. (U.S.)*, 54 (1965) 899.
141 D. R. Drury, *Am. J. Physiol.*, 131 (1940–41) 536.
142 D. Stetten and G. E. Boxer, *J. Biol. Chem.*, 156 (1944) 271.
143 J. Ganguly, *Biochim. Biophys. Acta*, 40 (1960) 110.
144 B. M. Waite and S. J. Wakil, *J. Biol. Chem.*, 237 (1962) 2750.
145 S. Numa, M. Matsuhashi and F. Lynen, *Biochem. Z.*, 334 (1961) 203.
146 A. F. Spencer and J. M. Lowenstein, *J. Biol. Chem.*, 237 (1962) 3640.
147 J. V. Formica, *Biochim. Biophys. Acta*, 59 (1962) 739.
148 D. W. Foster and B. Bloom, *Biochim. Biophys. Acta*, 70 (1963) 341.
149 W. M. Bortz and F. Lynen, *Biochem. Z.*, 339 (1963) 77.
150 K. Takeda and B. M. Pogell, *J. Biol. Chem.*, 241 (1966) 720.
151 P. K. Tubbs and P. B. Garland, *Biochem. J.*, 89 (1963) 25P.
152 H. M. Korchak and E. J. Mosoro, *Biochim. Biophys. Acta*, 58 (1962) 354.
153 O. Wieland and I. Eger-Neufeldt, *Biochem. Z.*, 337 (1963) 349.
154 W. M. Bortz, S. Abraham and I. L. Chaikoff, *J. Biol. Chem.*, 238 (1963) 1266.

155 C. A. PLATE, V. C. JOSHI, B. SEDGWICK AND S. J. WAKIL, *J. Biol. Chem.*, 243 (1968) 5439.
156 D. M. GIBSON AND D. D. HUBBARD, *Biochem. Biophys. Res. Commun.*, 3 (1960) 531.
157 O. WIELAND, I. EGEN-NEUFELDT, S. NUMA AND F. LYNEN, *Biochem. Z.*, 336 (1963) 455.
158 W. BENJAMIN AND A. GELHORN, *J. Biol. Chem.*, 239 (1964) 64.
159 D. W. ALLMANN, D. D. HUBBARD AND D. M. GIBSON, *J. Lipid Res.*, 6 (1965) 63.
160 S. NUMA, W. M. BORTZ AND F. LYNEN, *Advan. Enzyme Regulation*, 3 (1965) 407.
161 A. GELHORN AND W. BENJAMIN, *Science*, 146 (1964) 1166.
162 P. W. MAJERUS, personal communication (1969).
163 T. O. HENDERSON AND J. J. MCNEIL, *Biochem. Biophys. Res. Commun.*, 25 (1966) 662.
164 G. WEEKS AND S. J. WAKIL, *J. Biol. Chem.*, 245 (1970) 1913.
165 P. OVERATH, G. PAULI AND H. V. SCHAIRER, *Eur. J. Biochem.*, 7 (1969) 559.
166 G. WEEKS, M. SHAPIRO, R. O. BURNS AND S. J. WAKIL, *J. Bacteriol.*, 97 (1969) 827.
167 E. M. BARNES JR., A. C. SWINDELL AND S. J. WAKIL, *J. Biol. Chem.*, 245 (1970) 3122.
168 H. VAN DEN BOSCH AND P. R. VAGELOS, *Biochim. Biophys. Acta*, 218 (1970) 233.
169 C. A. PLATE, V. C. JOSHI AND S. J. WAKIL, *J. Biol. Chem.*, 245 (1970) 2868.
170 V. C. JOSHI, C. A. PLATE AND S. J. WAKIL, *J. Biol. Chem.*, 245 (1970) 2857.
171 F. LYNEN, D. OESTERHELT, E. SCHWEIZER AND K. WILLECKE, *Fed. Europ. Biochem. Soc., Proc. 4th Meeting, Oslo*, Academic Press, New York, 1968, p.1.
172 D. F. SILBERT, F. RUCH AND P. R. VAGELOS, *J. Bacteriol.*, 95 (1968) 1658.
173 M. ESFAHANI, E. M. BARNES JR. AND S. J. WAKIL, *Proc. Natl. Acad. Sci. (U.S.)*, 64 (1969) 1057.

SUBJECT INDEX

Acetate, ammonium salt, entry of mitochondrial matrix space, 37

Acetoacetate, formation from acetyl-CoA, β-hydroxy-β-methyl-glutaryl-CoA as intermediate, 91, 92

—, — —, in starvation and diabetes, 91, 92

— pathway, regeneration of CoA from acetyl-CoA and increased oxidation of FA in fasting and diabetes, 91, 92

Acetyl-CoA ACP transacylase, *E. coli*, acetyl-S-enzyme intermediate, 74

— —, —, incorporation of various acyl-CoA esters into FA, compared with their transacylation to ACP by —, (table), 75

— —, —, substrate specificity, 75

— carboxylase, activity during fasting, 94, 95

— —, allosteric control by citrate and isocitrate, 68, 94

— —, association with FA synthetase in the cytosol of the cell, 92

— —, biotin binding, 66, 67

— —, carboxybiotinyl enzyme formation, 67

— —, citrate activation, inhibition by malonyl-CoA, 95

— —, correlation between state of aggregation and level of enzyme activity, 70

— —, decrease in activity in prolonged starvation and diabetes, 97, 98

— —, electron microscopy, molecular dimensions, 70

— —, formation of carboxybiotinyl enzyme, 67

— —, free energy of cleavage of the CO_2–biotinyl–protein complex, 68

— —, malonyl-CoA formation, 67, 68

— —, mol. wt. of polymer and protomer, 69

— —, polymerization and depolymerization of enzyme molecule by citrate and isocitrate, 69, 94

Acetyl-CoA carboxylase, (*continued*)

— —, protomer, biotin content, 69

— —, —, dissociation into subunits by dodecyl sulphate, 69

— —, rate limiting in FA biosynthesis, 69, 94

— —, regulation through inhibition by long-chain acyl-CoA derivatives, 94

— —, stereospecificity of transfer of carboxyl group to acceptor, 68

—, levels in tissues, and diversion of pyruvate from oxidation to hexose synthesis, 16

—, metabolic substrates degraded to —, 18

— synthetase, substrates, mol. wt., requirement for K^+ and Mg^{2+}, 58

Acetyltransferase, in pyruvate dehydrogenase complex, formation of dihydrolipoate and acetyl-CoA, reversibility, 4

Aconitase, intracellular location, 24, 25

cis-Aconitate, ammonium salt, entry of mitochondrial matrix space, effect of phosphate and malate, 37, 39, 42

trans-Aconitate, ammonium salt, permeability of mitochondria, 37

ACP, *see* Acyl carrier protein

Acyl-ACP, as donor in acylation of L-α-glycerol phosphate in *E. coli* and *Cl. butyricum*, 80

—, utilization for complex lipid biosynthesis, 80

Acyl carrier protein, component analogous to *E. coli* ACP, in FA synthetase of pigeon liver, 83

—, — —, — of yeast, 81

—, *E. coli*, amino acid composition and sequence, 72, 73

—, —, density of charged side-chains at the surface of the molecule, 73

—, —, mol. wt., 73

—, —, physical properties, 71

[105]